How to Be a Care Consultant and Care Manager

Working With Elders and Their Families With Compassion and Respect

Joan McGinnis, MSW, LICSW
Gary E. Bloom, MS, LMFT

Published by Aging Well Press
Edmonds, Washington
agingwellpress.com

Printed in the U.S.A.
First printing 2019

Library of Congress Control Number:2019910742

ISBN: 978-1-7339993-0-4

Contents

For our parents: Marie, Eugene, Lisa, and Irwin

Foreword, by Brad Lancaster

You pick up books. You thumb. Mostly, you put the texts down and move along. Once in a while, you get lucky. Today, *you* are positively Irish.

The authors, Joan McGinnis and her spouse, Gary Bloom, are human treasure. By "treasure," I mean the sort of people you hunt persistently, but infrequently corner. Like the seldom-spotted Sasquatch, only real. If the world were a better place, Presidents would bestow more medals for extravagant care and fewer for martial sacrifice. One would glimpse Joan and Gary in the Oval Office, shy and squirming. Gary would pull at his necktie. Joan would elbow him. Each would duck a bit as the lanyard looped their necks. That non-existent award would gleam over their hearts, signaling America's gratitude. Sadly, we do not live in such an America. (But we should. We can work toward that.) Gary and Joan care—intelligently, persistently, sometimes without reward. If you seek mentorship as an elder care consultant or elder care manager, you are in luck. This is your book.

My opinion of the McGinnis-Bloom partnership is not promotional hyperbole, but a judgment of experience. I met Joan and Gary at a summer picnic of a mutual friend. We talked of law and elders and care challenges and the court system and guardianship and attorneys-in-fact. Gary's wry humor often cut; his intelligence is patent. Joan's technical insights were tinged with worldly wise affection. Beneath the ripple of laughter swept a current of compassion. The conversation made me glad to be alive, but it was just summer picnic jabber.

Then came Irene. Picnic talk became action. I had painted Irene's house, when I did that sort of thing for a living, before law school. Irene chose the ugliest color I ever applied in the many thousands of gallons of paint I brushed or sprayed (a puky green jumble of emerald, teal, and army). She decided that the bottom of her bottom siding board needed coating. So, I went around with a little mirror (I'd have had to dig a hole to get an eye so low) and dabbed the siding bottoms until all were covered. Her significant other, Robert, approved, feeling, in his penny-pinching Scottish bones, that Irene had gotten her money's worth. Irene and Robert attended our Fourth of July parties, annual bashes with a liberal slosh of alcohol for those so inclined. Robert and Irene imbibed and giggled.

One Independence Day, several years later, Robert took me aside. He asked me to draft end-of-life documents for him and Irene. I inquired. Robert was terminally ill. We hugged. More critical to Robert, Irene's mind was failing, a problem Robert had been tending (and concealing). Irene designated me her attorney-in-fact. And, upon Robert's sad passing, my odyssey with Irene began.

Irene's medical records revealed a complex set of issues: cardiac problems, and skin lesions, and dementia of unspecified origin. I called Joan McGinnis. Joan interviewed Irene. Joan offered analysis and created a care plan for Irene. I implemented Joan's plan. Joan managed the health care portion of Irene's needs, took Irene to her many medical appointments, and interfaced with the care providers at Irene's graduated care residential facility. Irene would utilize all the facility's care options before her end. Irene's mind was failing, but her sentiments were not. The woman lived with fierce independence. Every member of Irene's care team, at various points, skulked in the shadows to avoid offending Irene's need for perceived autonomy. She needed help, but accepted it, at best, reluctantly.

Near the beginning of these years, at Joan's suggestion, I hired a therapist who specialized in elders facing dementia. She met with Irene, mined Irene's memories, and wrote them down. She created a photographic album of Irene's past and gathered stories related to those persons with the images. These therapeutic work products helped keep Irene oriented, as brain dysfunction robbed her of life's landmarks.

Irene wandered. Many dementia patients wander. Irene, however, excelled. She never got lost unless she could not see the Space Needle. From its beacon, she could navigate to her residential facility. Paramedics transported Irene one night, lost, from a location fourteen miles distant. Another night, she disappeared. Concerned staff called me at 1:00 a.m. I jumped in my truck and drove Seattle's downtown alleys with my laptop. We found Irene's personal tracker in a dumpster (where she had thrown it). About 2:30 a.m., I sighted Irene tromping along the edge of Seattle Center, headed home. I gave her a lift. She had no explanation. Joan and Irene's care team met. Irene began bringing dead animals to the facility, even the dining room, seeking help for them. We moved Irene to assisted living, and after one last dangerous "adventure," to the dementia floor (with locked doors).

Irene had a friend, whom I will call Pandora, for she proved a nest of problems. Pandora suffered her own mental decline. She could neither accept Irene's changes nor appreciate their potential for danger. Pandora wanted their friendship to persist as though nothing had changed. Pandora took Irene driving; the two suffered collisions. She asked Irene to drink with her, which behavior improves dementia not the tiniest bit. She let Irene wander when inspiration struck. Irene tore her skin, which had grown fragile, a couple of times. More team meetings, which Joan led. We framed a plan for controlling and/or excluding Pandora from injuring Irene. The efforts proved marginally successful.

Irene's abilities flagged. She spent days bed-bound. She forgot all of us. But not her cat. Well, she forgot the cat's name. That feral animal bit me just because I was not Irene. When Irene left her space on the dementia floor, with elbow-length welding gloves, I captured that feline menace in its hiding place in the bathroom medicine cabinet, and delivered it to King County's animal shelter.

Irene's love of life ebbed, like a candle guttering. She stopped smiling and singing. She slowed, then stopped eating. Joan led the care team to a conclusion. We moved Irene to nursing care downstairs and called hospice. Our friend lay in bed for days. We tended her as we were able. Then one night, not so soon as mercy might have wished, Irene was gone.

Still, Joan's involvement was not complete. She helped me arrange to care for the grief of Irene's many friends, as well as our own. A memorial sang the ballad of such a life as Irene's, in words, in photos, in songs. Even in death, Irene made us glad to be alive.

So, that's my tale of care consultation and care management with Joan. The rewards of working for declining people are many, a few of which are, under the right circumstances, financial. Such persons long to be treated normally, though normalcy now eludes them. Are you a person who can listen under these sometimes-exigent circumstances? This book will help you, if you hear Irene's story and imagine yourself helping.

You could not have better teachers than Joan McGinnis and Gary Bloom.

Brad Lancaster
Shoreline, Washington
June 2019

Preface

If you were anything like me, when you were a child, you yearned to be a care consultant. You dressed in care consultant costumes on Halloween. You asked for care consultant outfits for birthday gifts, and you asked the multicultural gift-giver of your choice, sometime around the winter solstice, to deliver care consultant action figures. Your parents humored you, sure that you'd grow out of this fantasy, because when you were growing up, *there was no such thing as a care consultant!*

I began working with elders in 1984, but I didn't start calling myself a care consultant until a decade later. Even today, hardly anyone labels themselves as such, sticking with the well-known term, *care manager.* Yet, there is a significant difference between their roles. In short, a care consultant guides the concerned parties—usually, family members of the client (who is the elder, or otherwise, infirm)—to appropriate services. This typically requires a thorough assessment of the situation that includes the needs and wishes of the client, and an agreement among those involved in the care decisions—usually, the family. If the family is unable or uninterested in managing the care, they hire a care manager to do that. About one-third of the time that I'm hired for care consultation, I'm retained in the role of care manager.

While you may have guessed that I didn't really plan, let alone "yearn," to be a care consultant when I was young, I did plan to become a social worker. However, my work with elders was a fluke.

Before graduate school, I did some work in an inpatient hospital and became determined to work with the severely mentally ill. Following getting my MSW, I took a position working in a residential treatment center for chronic schizophrenics. During my five years there, I rose to program director. Moving on from that program, I followed my husband-to-be to a small town, where the only opening in the counseling center was as director of geriatric services. I was hired for my supervision experience, as I had no experience with elders.

My grad-school classmate and friend had been working with elders since her graduation. My agency agreed to pay for distance supervision, via phone calls. With her help, I managed my own work, supervised a nurse and clinician, and earned my state's recognition as a Geriatric Mental Health Specialist.

Unlike many non-fiction books, we couldn't have transformed a short book into a longer one by front-loading it with the history of the subject. We would have had too little to work with. The history of care consultation has less in common with a distinct profession and more in common with a town meeting led by whoever marched to the podium and grabbed the mic—usually a social worker, nurse, lawyer, wife, husband, sibling, daughter, or son. When the management of care of an elder is taken on by a professional—usually, a nurse or social worker—it's sometimes referred to as *case management* or the all-encompassing *care manager,* but these terms can mislead. Case management has a historical association with the mental health system and various social work, and care management is just an optional component of care consultation. I identify as a care consultant who sometimes gets hired to do care management.

Care consultation and care management training is often treated as a stepchild, by adding a certificate program or the like to a university department that studies and teaches geriatrics. But there is more to working with the elderly than understanding the aging process. Clinician-led care consultation and care management training is rare, and I believe it should be done by those with clinical training, whether in social work, counseling, or nursing.

The goal of this book is to create a source that can be used in a formal school setting or as a self-educational guide. It is not meant to be an instruction manual, but an offering, an invitation to what I've experienced and learned in my three-plus decades of working with the elderly. It's not meant to be an exhaustive reference but an aid to give you a head start, whether in private practice or within an agency.

This book was written by Joan McGinnis (me) and Gary Bloom. I'm a social worker who assembled a career as a care consultant during three decades. Gary is a marriage and family counselor, who has advised me on working with families. We happen to be married, which made this book both easier and harder to write.

Part I

The Care Manager

Chapter 1

The Care Manager

Recently, I spent several unanticipated hours attending to some basic needs of my client: was she fed, did she get her phone and TV installed?

She had just moved into a pricey assisted living facility, and during her first days there, had not received the services for which she was being charged. I ended up subsidizing the services of this facility by attending to these things, which meant that my client was paying me for what should have been taken care of by the facility.

I returned home, upset, and began to vent: "It's a good thing I'm detail-oriented, because those at the facility aren't!"

After listening to my frustration, my husband (co-author and go-to consultant) suggested that being detail-oriented is just a footnote to providing service. Service is being vigilant—alert to your clients' needs, sensitive to their moods. What needs to be done for them, detailed or not, follows from that.

That discussion got me to reflect on the difference between being detailed-oriented versus being sensitive to the needs of clients. A detail-oriented person (or efficiently run facility) would make sure that dinner was always served at 5 p.m., sharp. An individual (or facility) that was sensitive to the needs of clients would make sure their clients are not hungry. Being detail-oriented means every necessary service has been put in place. Being sensitive to the needs of clients means that you make sure those services are working for them. Being detailed-oriented means making sure meds are taken as prescribed. Being sensitive to clients' needs means that you observe the effects of those meds: are they helping, are they causing problems, or are they helping in some manner, but causing discomforting side-effects?

There are countless examples of the difference between being detail-oriented and being sensitive to the needs of clients, but in general, it boils down to this: being detail-oriented is about efficiency; being sensitive to the needs of clients is about service.[1]

The Responsibilities of the Care Manager

I could attempt to describe the profession of care management by listing common services that we provide, but as with any complex profession, being a care manager is not service by rote, and it's not a list of stuff we do, it's service guided by expertise and concern. The concern part comes from what I expressed above, being sensitive to clients' needs. That's necessary, the way fine-motor coordination for a surgeon, dentist, or mechanic is necessary. Expertise comes as always from experience and the training and education necessary to learn from experience.

A care manager is hired for several related reasons. Often, after a care consultant advises a family on the services that need to be put in place, the members of the family decide that they are too busy, or too much in conflict, or lack the confidence or skills to follow through on the initial or ongoing advice from the care consultant. Along with having knowledge of a wide variety of services, and knowing which ones will best serve a particular client, a care manager's main job is to get those

[1] Being detail-oriented often serves the needs of the person or agency providing the service more than it serves the needs of the client.

services to work in harmony. Though the required services might be practiced by skilled professionals—doctors, lawyers, nurses, accountants, physical therapists, social workers, counselors, placement specialists, assisted living facilities, and others—someone has to make sure these services work in harmony. And no matter how much family members, or otherwise concerned, care about the client, working with the various experts takes skill and experience. Let's look at some services a care manager might have to facilitate and/or coordinate:

- Doctor, dental, physical therapy and other health-care appointments
- Transition to an assisted living facility, hospital, nursing home
- Homecare services for clients who want to stay in their home
- Non-health professionals, such as lawyers, accountants, bill payers, attorney-in-fact

Along with the above services, the care manager will have to maintain agreed-upon communication with the client's family or designated family liaison.

An organized and compassionate person, even a healthcare professional, might think that he or she has all the skills and experience necessary to pull off being a care manager. He or she might, but the training and experience necessary to communicate effectively with all the various people and agencies mentioned above (and there are more), might be beyond the experience and expertise of a professional in another field. Care management is a challenging professional field that requires compassion, specific training, and specific clinical experience.[2]

[2]The training and experience of many healthcare professionals still leave out many of the services I routinely address with my clients.

Your Training

In my state of Washington, and many others, if you apply eyeliner to someone's face for money, you need a license from the state. If you paint someone's nails for money, you need a license from the state. I have no doubt this is a good thing, as applying cosmetics or working with utensils on delicate hands can result in infections. Still, coordinating care among doctors, rehabilitation agencies, care facilities, counselors, lawyers, dentists, money handlers, transportation providers, and other care providers to the elderly and infirm—and doing it, badly—can result in problems far worse. Yet, anyone can call themselves a care manager and charge money for their services.

I certainly don't believe that the right to care for loved ones should be regulated, but at the same time, I believe adopting care management as a profession should require at least as much training and regulation as painting nails for money. I'll go on a limb and say, I think care management as a profession should require even more training than painting nails and applying eyeliner.[3]

If your work with elders and their families goes beyond managing care, that is, it includes comprehensive advice on what services are necessary to sustain health and well being, you have crossed the boundary into care consultation. Poor advice, at this level, can result in costly, unnecessary, or even harmful choices for care. Just as advice from a good medical, legal, or financial professional, advice from a good care consultant should result in better *and* less costly care in the long run.

Your career as a care consultant should benefit your clients and benefit you as a professional. And that requires a combination of education, training, and experience. (Care consultation is covered in Part III, Screening and Assessments, and Part IV, Working With Families.)

[3]No disrespect to cosmeticians and manicurists, intended.

Paths to a Career

A devoted family member can be an effective care manager to a loved one. She or he may be in a position to devote an unusual amount of time to one person: They can spend countless hours accompanying the elder to necessary appointments, assertively question medical personnel on treatment plans, research options on the Internet, involve lawyers and other professionals as needed, discuss options with involved family members, and deal with other tasks that may arise.

My concern is that those whose care management experience comes primarily from managing a single individual will not be prepared to deal with the immense variety of client issues that come with a significant-sized clientele. Furthermore, when faced with new situations that are often frighteningly complex, many fall back on seeing everything as a scrapbook because their only tool is a glue stick. Your elderly mother is not the prototype for every client.

After many years of practice, I still deal with novel situations, many are complex novel situations. Even with my warehouse of experience, I can't always fall back on knowledge learned from specific clients. What I can fall back on is that I've learned to deal with new challenges. And so have you, from playing in the sandbox as a child, to negotiating advanced education, relationships, and jobs. You've learned to use experience, mentors (primarily in the form of parents, older siblings, and teachers), and knowledge gained from media, all of which you use to negotiate new challenges.

To learn care management and care consultation, you'll again want to combine learning from mentors, formal education, and experience. How to best do this is in flux. Professionally trained care managers primarily come from backgrounds in social work, counseling, and nursing. All three of these professions have the sort of involvement with the wide world of health care and of the legal system that can prepare you for care consultation/management. And all three have their advantages and disadvantages.

Nurses, of course, will be most attuned to health issues, highly useful to clients with ongoing health problems. Their systemic experience and knowledge will be weighted towards health care.

Counselors will be most experienced in dealing with emotional issues and problems in mental health that often accompany new infirmities or death of a spouse (or partner).

Social workers are trained in what most constitutes care management, acting as an advocate for the client and as intermediary among the members of the treating and familial system. As a social worker, until there are more dedicated clinical care management and care consultation training programs, I advise that, if you are certain you want to go into care management and care consultation, and you're not yet trained in nursing or counseling, start your training with social work.

That said, good care managers come from backgrounds in nursing and counseling, and the above descriptions of professional training are generalizations. For example, social workers and nurses may also have extensive training and experience in the mental health field. Regardless of your particular training, the most important attributes of a care manager/consultant are a dedication to learning, a systemic focus, and a genuine sensitivity to the needs of your clients.

Part II

The Client's Experience

Chapter 2

Old Age and Loss

Getting old isn't for wimps.
—Unknown

Joe Montana, one of the most accomplished professional athletes of all time, played into his late 30s. He was asked—with four Super Bowl victories and two most valuable player awards, but at the cost of accumulated injuries—why he kept playing? His answer: "What if someone told you that you will never get to do again what you love the most?"

Moving into old age brings a series of all the things you'll never get to do again: loved ones you'll never see again; ideas your mind will no longer be able to contemplate no matter how smart you once were; places, such as your beloved home, that you'll never live in again; memories you'll never have again; social status you'll never enjoy again; and for many, the biggest insult of all, personal independence you'll never have again. Getting old is an insult to your self-esteem, to your physical comfort, to your identity as an adult. No wonder the elderly yell at folks to get off their lawn.

It's not all bad: young grandchildren to spoil, then home to their parents to deal with the consequences; no dreary job to go to or worry about being laid off; cheap health care; discounts; for some, fewer financial worries; less need for shopping, as you probably have enough clothes to last your lifetime; you've bought your last car, your last home, and last pair of Nike Jordans; failures forgotten, successes enhanced.

If you describe the elderly as cute, intolerant, dumb with technology, or other condescending labels, think again. We find young children cute because they're innocent of most of life's experiences. By definition, older people have more life experiences than younger people. Intolerant? Everyone is more comfortable with the world in which they grew up because they're experts in negotiating that world. Same for technology. Familiar is easier, but don't forget, older people dealt with less automated machines, less technology that (to borrow from the old Apple motto) just worked. Telling Siri to place a phone call does not make you more clever than those who dialed rotary phones for much of their lives.

To say that old people don't like change is silly. With decades behind them, most older people have survived many downs and have a long history of adapting to change. They just don't like turns for the worse any more than anyone else does, and they've had more of those than have most younger people. And those turns for the worse will continue. In more detail, as you get older, you must adapt to numerous unpleasant changes:

Loss of family
Loss of friends
Loss of vision
Loss of hearing
Loss of mobility
Loss of memory
Loss of independence as in the ability to drive, care for self, etc.
A shrinking support system
Decreased abilities
Fewer choices

Decreased activity
Decreased socializing

That's a lot of losses. Getting old isn't for wimps.

Chapter 3

Why Are They Doing This to Me?

Rose is a 78-year-old woman living alone in her condominium. To family, friends, and neighbors, she seems to be doing well. She is in good health and remains physically and socially active. Her adult children call her "bright" and note her continuous interest in reading and current events. She views herself as competent and independent and is proud of her intellect.

Rose begins to notice that her keys aren't where she recalls leaving them. She is uncertain if she paid her phone bill and can't find her checkbook. She leaves a pan of soup on the stove until she is alarmed by the smell of burnt food. She forgets a lunch date with a friend.

No big deal. She finds her keys. She finds her checkbook. She pays her phone bill. She throws out the burned pan. She apologizes to her friend and schedules another lunch date.

Although the forgetful incidents continue, Rose doesn't mention it; there's nothing to discuss. She doesn't want her children to think she needs help, and she's not interested in making changes. Nevertheless, the burned pan worries her, so she stops preparing meals and turns to snacking. No big deal, she's never had a big appetite.

Rose is distressed, however, when she notices she can no longer follow a novel to the end. She forgets who the characters are and begins to get confused about their motivations. Nothing like this has ever happened to her. And still, she tells no one. She is competent, independent, and intelligent.

Unfortunately, Rose's poor nutrition makes her vulnerable to illness, and she catches pneumonia. She is hospitalized and a dramatic change in her behavior is observed. She doesn't want to take prescribed medications and tries to leave the hospital. She is transferred to the geropsychiatric unit, and an evaluation determines that she has deterioration of the brain consistent with dementia. Once Rose is stabilized on calming medications, she's transferred to a nursing home that has a secured dementia unit.

Rose had been experiencing gradual cognitive decline but did a good job of hiding it. Eventually, she underwent a rapid decline and accompanying change in behavior that required medical intervention.

To understand Rose, let's step inside her head. You're living on your own and have tricked yourself into believing that the changes you see in yourself do not require changes in your day-to-day life. You continue to be proud of your intellect and competence and want to be damn sure that others are proud of you too, especially your children.

You get sick and delirious. Medical professionals you don't know and have no reason to trust are giving you pills and preventing you from leaving. You want to go back to your condo and resume the life you enjoy. And you desperately want to get back to your old self, the self you are proud of. There is nothing familiar about this place, nothing that reminds you of who you are. You're surrounded by people—doctors, nurses, aides—who are in-your-face with their ignorance of who you are.

Take your medications. You have to stay here. No, you can't leave. We're just trying to help you.

They see you as sick and suffering, unappreciative and uncooperative. They have no idea who you are, who you have been. They do not know your story. They do not see you.

And then you are in a secured (locked) unit. You have never had to wonder what was beyond a door. You just walked to it, opened it, and walked to the other side. And your mind, your innate intelligence, has allowed you to open many figurative doors to other worlds. Now, an all-too-real door is closed to you.

Now I ask, wouldn't you want to go out that door?

Chapter 4

The Loss of the Ability to Communicate Makes You a Ghost

"✻" Denotes the beginning of an example.

The eleventh episode of *Buffy the Vampire Slayer,* "Out of Mind, Out of Site,"[1] is about a high school girl who, because no one at school pays attention to her, gradually transforms into a ghost. In Chapter 2, I list the many losses the elderly face. Along with the loss of health and loved ones, as belonging to the most social of species, the worst loss is the ability to communicate with others. Our greatest social desire is to express ourselves and be understood, and the elderly may face a number of setbacks in their ability to understand and be understood.

✻ Diane is an artist who loves faces and the movement of the human body. She remarks on color, shapes, nature, and anything else in her field of vision. We sit in the lobby of where she lives, and she comments

[1]https://en.wikipedia.org/wiki/Out_of_Mind,_Out_of_Sight_(Buffy_the_Vampire_Slayer)?wprov=sfsi1)

on the beauty of those who come through the door. "Oh! Look at her gorgeous red curls." "Isn't her scarf a beautiful color?" "What a lovely smile!"

She describes a top I'm wearing, "It's like running up the stairs!" Another day, another top. "It's like being under water."

Diane suffers from dementia. She answers direct questions indirectly and is unable to recall enough of her life to tell a consistent history. She flits from one topic to another. To improve my relationship with her and my recommendations about her care, I must weave the fragments she reveals into a tale of her identity.

* Anna punctuates her discourse with "I've lost my words."[2] Or, she substitutes inaccurate words for words she means. Each conversation is a challenge to guess her meaning.

Anna lives in a dementia care facility and is troubled by the loss of independence. She resists assistance from care givers. She tells me, "I hate it here. I want to leave." When I ask what she dislikes about living there, she is unable to explain. My challenge is to figure out how she would answer my questions if she could—a game of Clue far harder than the board game. The clues are limited to what I know about her history and what I observe in her interactions with me and others.

* George attempting to explain: "There are a lot of parts to this and stuff related to going here, or going there. It's not just do this, it's there's a lot to it, and a lot of work to sort through all of it. And there are different people here and there, and how long it takes to get to one or the other. With one it's just go here, and there's the stuff that I do before and with someone. There's a lot more time and work I have to do and parts to this."

Throughout his attempt to communicate, he gestures and when finished looks at me, as if to ask, "Do you understand?"

[2]Clinically, it's called trouble with *word finding*.

George began to suffer from primary progressive aphasia at a relatively young age. In trying to convey his experience of having to make a major change—he's been looked after by a companion/care giver during the day and now is attending an adult day center—all he can do is express himself in generalities. I understand that he's overwhelmed and anxious, and the "parts" he refers to are unclear to him. What is clear to him is that a change in his routine has been necessary, and change is difficult for someone with cognitive impairment. My task is to break the issue down into parts he can understand.

As a consultant to nursing homes, I led group therapy for elders who were struggling with depression, anxiety, and dementia. In one of these groups, a participant began to tell a story about a train trip she took as a teenager. Being new to this group, I noticed the rolling eyes and glazed looks on the faces of other group members. To allay the boredom and contempt, I had to help this woman expand upon her story—a tale she had obviously told, repeatedly—while inviting others to talk about their experiences on trains. Often-repeated stories hold profound meaning for a person suffering from dementia. These stories convey a part of their character or experience that defines who they have been in the world and who they still are.

When communicating with someone with memory loss, word finding difficulty, tangentiality, aphasia, or any communication disability, I observe all the non-verbal clues I can and convey what I hear and understand.

✻ At one point in our conversation, Anna says with a surprised tone, "You understand me." And near the end of another conversation that's rich with emotion, she says, "You have this box, and you take things from it." She makes the shape of a box and makes gestures of lifting things from it, one by one. I take this to mean that I store my understanding of her in a metaphorical box and communicate parts of it back to her to help her understand the painful emotions she's experiencing.

Whether I tease out the meaning of repeated stories, read body language, weave the story of a life from disjointed sentences, obtain a gestalt of meaning from a bunch of words, or store my understanding in a metaphorical box, I create a bridge to communicate about their experience of the world. These efforts are appreciated by those who need badly to be understood.

Chapter 5

Religion and Spirituality

For clients whose religious or spiritual life is important, I help them continue with their religious or spiritual center of choice. Occasionally, this means I have contact with their minister, priest, rabbi, or other cleric.

My level of assistance varies. When a client was temporarily or permanently homebound, I coordinated visits from Eucharist ministers. I've coordinated transportation to religious services. I have helped clients find living facilities that offered their preferred religious services.

I've had a single opportunity to work directly with a priest. A client's attorney-in-fact (AIF) wanted the Physician's Orders for Life Sustaining Treatment (POLST) to be consistent with guidelines of the Catholic Church. To ensure this consistency, my client, his AIF, and I met with their priest, who stayed involved when my client was admitted to hospice for end-of-life care.

On rare occasions, clients have asked about my religious or political leanings. I explain that my work is not tied to either a religious or political affiliation, but that their faith and spiritual life is relevant to my work in the role that it plays in their life.

I have yet to lose a client over religious or political issues.

Part III

Screening and Assessments

Chapter 6

Screening and Intake

Initial Screening Phone call

I offer a twenty-minute call to potential clients. The screening deals with the following questions: (1) Who's the client? (2) Do I provide the services the caller is seeking? (3) Am I currently accepting new clients for the services the caller is seeking? (4) Are the services being sought likely to be consultation, ongoing care management, or both? And, after these questions are answered, if the caller wishes to proceed (5) who will be the billable party? (6) Who will be at the initial consultation, and why?

Obviously, getting new clients is good for business; I like to eat as much as the next person. Nevertheless, I consider screening mutually beneficial. There are reasons I may or may not want to take on a client, and there are reasons they may not want to hire me.

I might be too busy in either the short term or the long term to provide the services they need. If their needs can wait, and they're still interested, I'll tell them to get back to me at a future date.

When the services I provide don't match what they're seeking, I'll refer them to other services.

Who's the client?

Identifying the client should be straightforward.[1] The client is the person who's in need of care and/or planning for their future care. Typically, the initial contact is with the adult child, whose parent(s) may be suffering from the onset of cognitive impairment, a physical ailment for which they need ongoing care, or a number of other difficulties related to aging. I inform the caller that, regardless of who pays my bill, my recommendations are based solely on the client's needs for current and future care.[2] I also make it clear that I consider the client's financial resources, and my first consideration is to not add to a client's problems.

The message that my sole concern is with the needs of the client alerts callers that, regardless of their assumptions, my focus will be on their parent (or in some cases, parents). I say this up front, because while uncommon, adult children may have an unspoken conflicting interest. Why unspoken? That can range from secret conflicts with other family members to adult children who care more about their inheritance than the well-being of their parent. (I discuss this further in Chapter 7, How Things Go Wrong.) Most often, my message puts callers at ease: "I'm so glad to hear that. It's exactly what I was hoping for."

There are occasional exceptions to the identified client being the person in need of service. (See Chapter 18, Who's the Client?) A lawyer may contract with me for a narrative assessment of his or her client or to research a specific topic. (See Chapter 21, Lawyers.) Or a guardian may hire me to perform a specific task. (See Chapter 26, Guardians.)

When callers ask about my background, experience, and services, it may indicate that they're researching options. I don't bother to sell myself. In the long run, people defend their careful choices but grow resentful when they've felt manipulated. I show my expertise through

[1]Identifying the client should be straightforward, but can be confusing. See Chapter 18, Who's the Client?

[2]Because it's an issue that comes up more often than most, I emphasize that repeatedly in this book.

pointed questions. After we've both gone through our questions, I refer them to my website for additional information.

Callers' questions suggest what services they're seeking. If the questions are vague and/or anxious, I seek clarification: why are they seeking help and why now? If they're dealing with a crisis, I decide if I can help or if they need a referral to an emergency service. They can contact me if they still want my services after the emergency has been dealt with.

For example, to a caller who describes an elderly family member who's suffered a fall and displays confusion, my first question is, "Has this been reported to the primary physician?" If the answer is no, after discussing the issues and obtaining the caller's contact information, I advise they call the primary physician for a medical assessment.

Why I might turn down potential clients

I might turn down clients if they're not within my practice focus, or are outside my comfort zone, or are unmanageable within my current caseload.

Early in my career, I decided I would not supervise other service providers, such as private care givers who are hired by a client or their family. Because I'm not the private care givers' employer, I'm unwilling to assume responsibility for the quality of their service. For example, if a caller wants to hire someone to set up and oversee 24-hour home care, I refer them to an agency that provides those services.

Further examples of who I refer out are those who exhibit signs of dementia and paranoia while having access to guns and those who use illegal drugs. In the former case, I would accept them if the firearms were removed. In the latter case, I would refer them to a drug counselor.

As a sole practitioner, when screening referrals, I must keep in mind my workload. If I'm devoting many hours to ongoing care-management clients, I limit new clients to those who need only brief consultation.

These are lines I draw. Based on your expertise and the evolution of your practice, you'll have to define your limits and limitations.

Consultation, or ongoing management of care?

When someone calls to discuss my services, they usually have an idea of what they want. They may not be able to state that they want consultation or that they want management, but I can often determine that during the screening. If they're undecided, the decision can wait until our first meeting.

Who will be the billable party?

I determine the billable party before the initial consultation. I refer the caller to my service agreement and disclosure on my website. If there's a question who will pay the bill, I ask the caller to resolve that issue before the initial appointment. Most often, the spouse or the adult child who's the *attorney-in-fact* (AIF)[3] for the client assumes payment responsibility.

Who will be at the initial consultation and why?

I may ask that the client be excluded from the initial consultation. If the client suffers from dementia, it can be stressful if the cognitive status and need for care are discussed in the client's presence.

At times, the AIF may bring up whether the client should or shouldn't participate in the initial consultation. If they don't bring it up, I do. I want to gather information without causing stress to my client.

Intake and the Intake Form

This section describes the nuts and bolts of intake. Involvement and negotiation with the family are covered in *Part VI, Working with Families*.

[3]The AIF is often called the *agent*, and they are often inaccurately called the *durable power of attorney*, which is actually the name of a document, rather than the person. We will use the term attorney-in-fact or AIF for short. Also, note that the AIF is seldom an attorney.

I ask my client or their representative to bring a copy of their durable power of attorney (DPOA). This document identifies the representative as a decision-making authority—*the attorney-in-fact*—for the client. In addition, I ask that they provide the client's diagnoses and a list of current prescribed medications.

During the balance of the meeting, we clarify the client's issues (the reasons I'm being consulted), make an agreement on the services I will provide, and I collect the information necessary to provide these services.

Demographic information

I begin with the basics: date services are initiated; date of revisions;[4] name, date of birth, age, sex, marital status, address, phone number(s); client lives alone or with others; medical insurance;[5] preferred hospital.

Presenting problem/identified needs

I note what problems and needs my client, or my client's representative, identify.

Care plan

I write a brief summary of the plan I will assist my client with. This is helpful if specific actions will be taken soon.

Emergency contacts, AIFs, and involved parties

Emergency contacts includes the names, relationship to the client, phone numbers, and emails of individuals my client has given me permission to communicate with regarding my client's status and care. There is likely to be an overlap with the client's AIF(s) for medical and financial decision-making.

Involved parties may include homecare agencies, private care givers, bill payers, financial advisers, housekeepers, and close friends who

[4]With ongoing care management, I often complete a new intake form when significant changes or additions are made.

[5]Medicare, or other, I restate that my services are not covered by insurance

provide care or support. Involved parties may also include a visiting pastor, Eucharistic minister, priest, rabbi, or wellness practitioners such as a meditation coach or masseuse.

Medical information

I record diagnoses; medications including over-the-counter drugs, vitamins and supplements; and name and contact information of their primary physician. I record medical history when relevant to current care. If I'm to provide care management, I need the names and contact information of involved physicians. I record the names of additional medical services such as physical, occupational, or speech therapy.

I note assistive devices (cane, walker, wheelchair, medical alert button), or if my client wears glasses or a hearing aid, or uses a pill box to help with taking medications.

If I will be managing my client's care and attending medical appointments, I may need the pharmacy contact information.

Additional information

I record information that does not fit in the above categories: the client's faith, cultural background, sexual orientation; ongoing involvement in a service organization, and a relevant education or work history.

The referral source

Who referred the client to me?

Chapter 7

How Things Go Wrong

If you're from my generation, when you applied for jobs, you nearly always fielded the question, *what are your weaknesses?* You were taught to finesse it by turning your so-called weaknesses into strengths: *I work too hard,* or *I'm too self-critical*—answers that reeked of baloney. But fair is fair. With a job on the line, are you going to be candid? *I'm kind of lazy,* or, *I rarely know what I'm doing. I had to resign from my last job before they caught on.*

The job interviewer didn't deserve an honest answer.[1] But it's not just a näive question, it's also an ignorant one. What we think of as a weakness in ourselves (and others) is the flip side of what we characterize as our strengths. Our personalities aren't plucked from a smorgasbord of healthy preferences, they're a fixed-price meal—for better or worse, the courses go together. For example, if you're the type who's zealously devoted to the well-being of your clients, your empathy may stretch to giving everyone the benefit of the doubt. That emotional generosity may be laudable under many circumstances but can blunt your perceptions.

To get specific, you may have missed the hints that you haven't been hired to do what's best for the elder, you've been hired to do the dirty

[1]Imagine the job seeker asking, "What sucks about your company?"

work for a family member. So when conflict arises, it stems from hearing what you want to hear, not from what's been said.

If my consultation is going badly, it's likely that the unspoken motivation during that first phone call is that I was hired to do a specific thing that would benefit the caller rather than the client. It could be about money, for example, a concern that I might recommend services that would benefit the client but reduce a future inheritance. It could be about getting the elder out of the caller's hair; they want me to help them place the elder somewhere against the elder's wishes. It could be an attempt to get me to side with the caller's wishes over that of another family member.

Since it's rarely above-board, how will you know a conflict is stirring? Here's been my experience: Though I take great efforts to keep my costs as low as possible, the disappointed family member begins to make petty complaints about my bill. Or I start to receive subtle or not-so-subtle hostile remarks in emails that don't seem to match my efforts with the client.

When dealing with family complaints, my knee-jerk reaction is to defend my work. How I should respond, and eventually get to, is suggest we may have some misunderstandings, and we should renegotiate my role. In that renegotiation, I want to learn what was left unsaid during our initial conversations. Commonly, because I'm unwilling to work against the best interests of my client, this leads to the dissolution of our contract.

I leave these situations frustrated, but I accept these conflicts as my fault. I have a responsibility to make initial agreements as clear as possible, and at the first hint that there's conflict regarding my role, either renegotiate or end my role.

While conflict between a client's needs and the desires of an involved relative is commonly unsolvable, that's not always the case. The only way to find out is to renegotiate my role. For me, getting comfortable with that is an ongoing lesson.

Finally, I want to be clear that these conflicts are rare. In my years as a care consultant and care manager, nearly every family member of my clients has been honest and candid and want what's best for a loved one.

Chapter 8

Types of Assessments

I'll define three types of assessments, but in practice, these categories overlap. Care consultation is not routine, which is why this is a guide not a manual. Here are the following types of assessments:

A one-off written assessment. On occasion, a client's attorney-in-fact (AIF) or lawyer will request, as my only service, a comprehensive written assessment. Written assessments may be used to resolve disputes regarding care for those who no longer have the capacity to make their own medical and financial decisions.

An assessment for recommendations and referrals. Involvement with the client and/or decision maker(s) for the client is time-limited. The focus is on providing recommendations and referrals to address current care needs and develop a road map for future care.

An assessment and ongoing involvement with the client. Once information is obtained for the initial assessment, additional information is gathered over time. Recommendations are updated when there are changes in medical status and care needs.

Chapter 9

Introduction to Ongoing and Brief Assessments

In healthcare services, assessments are nearly always done on a standard form or form framework that's designed to satisfy health insurance requirements. As a practitioner, I find these forms too generic; they're designed to serve the agency rather than the clients.

A comprehensive written assessment takes 10 to 15 hours, and although it may provide a useful framework for future care, it rarely suits any urgent concerns.

In the bad news/good news department, there's no insurance coverage for care consultation, so if you're in private practice or don't work for an agency that requires a standard form, you won't have to use something that doesn't serve your clients. If you do work in an agency that uses a standard intake assessment, you may have to augment that with something that you'll find more applicable.

When I was the Director of Care Management at an agency, we had a contract with a crisis clinic to provide consultation to care givers—usually a family member or spouse[1] of an elder. The crisis typically arose

[1] By spouse, I mean legally married, or in current vernacular, *partner*.

because the elder was suffering from one or more problems, such as dementia, anxiety, depression, or disability.

The elder suffering from dementia might be (1) failing to take medications as prescribed, (2) wandering at night, (3) "losing" her car, (4) getting into minor traffic accidents. The elder may be suffering or is at risk for falls in a home that hasn't been adapted to that risk. The elder may be suffering from depression that results in social isolation and failure to maintain adequate nutrition. The elder may be refusing outside help that results in an unsustainable burden to the care givers.

The contract with the Crisis Clinic limited my services to ten hours per client. With that limit peering over my shoulder and tapping its feet, impatiently, I developed an efficient assessment process. I would meet with the care giver, on occasion the elder, at times hold a meeting that included other family members, and assess financial and other resources. Finally, I assembled a plan to address current and future needs and made recommendations.

As a private practitioner, I'm not constrained to complete services within ten hours, but my work with the Crisis Clinic taught me to be sensitive to both the time and financial constraints of a particular situation. I have carried that mindset with me. In all three assessment types, I begin with obtaining information about the client and the care system, quickly and efficiently. An example from each of the three categories of assessments, follows.

When There Will Not Be Ongoing Care Consultation or Care Management

Gathering information

* John contacts me and explains that his 89-year-old father, Harold, has been diagnosed with dementia six years ago. A retired college professor,

Harold is intelligent and has many interests and hobbies. However, his dementia is advancing to the point where he is unable to perform simple tasks to assist his wife, Dorothy. As she has to correct his errors, his attempts to help her have become a burden. For example, Harold has always sorted their trash for recycling, but is no longer capable. In addition, his favorite hobby, gardening, presents a risk to him. Harold has always pruned the trees and maintained the landscaping, but it is no longer safe for him to prune the trees that require he climb a ladder.

Finally, John and Dorothy feel that it's unsafe for Harold to be left alone. Harold's belief that he's still able to engage in simple activities, such as making tea or taking a walk by himself, puts him at risk.

Initial questions:

- Who is the AIF for the identified client?
- Who will attend the consultation?
- Who will pay for my services?
- Will Harold be involved in the consultation? Why or why not?

John explains that Dorothy, who is Harold's AIF, will contract for my services. We agree that Dorothy and John (who is the successor, i.e., the back up AIF for both parents) will attend the office consultation. We also agree it's best not to include Harold in the consultation, since discussion of concerns related to his advancing dementia could be both confusing and embarrassing.

John and Dorothy want to provide care for Harold in the home as long as possible and support Harold's independence as much as possible, while protecting him from harm. John confirms this approach reflects his father's wishes.

To enable completion of the assessment of Harold's needs and of Dorothy's need for support as his primary care giver, we discuss these questions:

- Does Dorothy manage Harold's prescribed medications, if any, and/or provide any other personal care assistance?
- Does Dorothy have health issues of her own?
- Are any housekeeping or yard-maintenance services currently in place?
- Are any caregiving services currently in place?
- What help is provided by the (three) adult children?
- Is the help provided by the adult children a burden to them? If so, can some or all of that assistance be contracted out?
- Are transportation needs safely addressed?
- Is the home environment conducive to care?
- Has either Harold or Dorothy suffered any falls in or around the home?
- When alone, does Harold ever leave a burner on, wander from the home, or do anything one might consider unsafe?
- Does Dorothy feel she has sufficient respite from caregiving responsibilities?

Conclusion

I followed our meeting with an email to Dorothy and John, summarized the situation, and made recommendations to best use current paid services and family help. I also provided references to homecare services for future needs.

When There Will Be Ongoing Involvement in Care Consultation

Gathering information

* Paul, one of three children of an elderly couple, calls with concerns regarding the safety of his parents. His father has had multiple hospital-

izations within the past year, most preceded by a fall. Mother has also been recently hospitalized and was discharged with medication changes.

Paul explains that his father frequently seeks medical attention for several concerns that don't get resolved or even clarified. Father has recently been diagnosed with dementia. Although Paul and his mother have seen evidence of memory loss, his father is not persuaded.

Paul states that his parents disagree whether to remain in their home or move to assisted living. Father prefers to remain in their home and expects his wife to take on increasing responsibility for his daily care and their household; Mother wants to move—yesterday. According to Paul, father calls the shots. Paul contacts me for help to devise a plan, first with getting care in the home, then with a move to assisted living.

Initial questions, logistical:

- Who will sign the service agreement and disclosure statement to initiate services?
- Who is/are the decision makers?
- Have Paul's parents assigned attorney-in-fact (AIF) to each other, with one or two of their children as the successor (back-up) AIFs?
- Are medical and financial AIFs held by the same or different individuals?
- Are the other adult children involved? If so, how?
- Who will attend the initial consultation or assessment?
- Where will the initial consultation or assessment take place—in my office or in their home, and why?

Further questions:

- What are Paul's parents' medical diagnoses and prescribed medications?
- Do they take medications as prescribed and follow all medical recommendations?
- Why is the father falling and being hospitalized frequently?

- Is the home more than one level? Must they take stairs to living and/or sleeping areas?
- Why was Paul's mother hospitalized?
- What care for her husband does she provide, and is her health being affected by providing it?
- In addition to the stress, what risks are there to mother in caring for her husband?
- Why do they disagree on whether to remain in their home or move to an assisted living facility?
- Have they enlisted any in-home help in the past; if they have, why was it discontinued?
- Do family members provide any assistance?
- Do the parents have friends who provide social and/or emotional support?

Conclusion

Because his parents disagree whether to enlist home care or move to an assisted living facility, the first step is an office consultation with their son and AIF, Paul. In the consultation, most of the above questions are answered. Following our meeting, we schedule a home assessment.

When There Will Be Ongoing Involvement in Care Management

Gathering information

* An adult daughter, who lives out of state, is concerned about her father's care and the stress her father's (second) wife is undergoing to provide that care. Her father is over 90, and her stepmother is in her late 80s. The daughter reports that her father suffers from dementia and impaired mobility and has experienced recent falls and weight loss. On her behalf and her three siblings (also out of state), the daughter

hires me to do an assessment and to provide care management services to their father.

At times, I must determine the AIF before I can provide services, and the determination in this case was not immediately obvious.

The brother of the daughter who contacted me (i.e., my client's son) has been his father's AIF before his father remarried. His children are concerned that their father's new wife had a lawyer transfer the AIF from the son to herself. They're alarmed because she also is showing signs of cognitive decline. She appears confused about the couple's finances, has let some bills go unpaid, and is overwhelmed with her role as her husband's care giver. None of these indicators bode well for her assuming responsibility as their father's AIF.

The daughter and her siblings are also worried that their stepmother makes a lengthy freeway drive for their father's medical care at the Veterans Administration Medical Center (VA).

Initial questions:

- What are my client's diagnoses and medications?
- Will the client or AIF sign a release of information to allow me to exchange information with the VA?
- Is my client eating balanced meals? How is his appetite? Has there been a change in appetite, and if so, has this been reported to his primary care physician? Has a weight loss been reported to, or noted by, his primary care physician?
- How frequently do my client and his wife visit the VA for his medical care?
- Where, and how often, do the reported falls occur?
- Have all falls been reported to my client's primary care physician?
- What is the bathing set-up, and who assists with bathing?
- How much help in transfer assistance does my client require?
- What mobility aides are used: walker, wheelchair, or cane?

- Has a home safety evaluation been completed by a physical therapist? If so, how recently, and what are the recommendations?
- Is the VA providing any homecare services to my client or support services for his wife as his care giver?

Questions that were answered over time:

- Who holds AIF for my client?
  Although his wife reported that she had changed AIF to herself, it was determined that AIF was still held by his son.

In addition, the following questions were eventually answered:

- What transportation services are available through the VA?
- What homecare services are available through the VA?
- What caregiver support services are available through the VA?

Conclusion

When you have been hired to do ongoing care management, the assessment is also ongoing. As needs arise or change, so do your recommendations and referrals. For example, in this situation, I eventually help coordinate the couple's move to an assisted living facility.

Chapter 10

Introduction to the Comprehensive Written Assessment

Before I was a care consultant, I was a counselor at a residential treatment center for chronic schizophrenics. I worked side-by-side with about 15 residents, sharing common daily tasks we called *life-skills practice*, and met weekly with the two or three residents who were my primary responsibility.

In addition to face-to-face counseling with my primary residents, I was required to write an assessment based on the information found in their charts that documented their histories in the mental health system. Most had experienced their first schizophrenic break when in their late teens or early twenties. They were now in their late twenties to mid-thirties and had undergone multiple hospitalizations.

I detested writing these assessments. I found it painful to stuff their complex three-dimensional lives into a two-dimensional assessment. Many of our residents were intelligent, some extremely so, and before their first psychotic episode, had been talented musicians or artists. Their multiple hospitalizations, treatment with anti-psychotic drugs, and stays (voluntary and involuntary) at various treatment centers, had robbed them of choices to pursue their talents, let alone employ them in a career. Writing about their lives laid bare lost opportunities and forecast hopeless futures.

Worst of all, in addition to being time-consuming and painful, and in my mind of little value to my work with clients, these assessments took me away from the point of being there, working with the residents.

The value of a care consultant is to respond to your client's specific needs as they change over time and to help them maintain the highest level of independence and the best quality of life possible, given their financial means and network of support. The static document you create for a specific request, for a specific circumstance, does not create a rich three-dimensional description of your client. The comprehensive written assessment (CWA) does little to support my work, and I undertake it when only specifically requested.

Almost all the CWAs I've done have been from a request from my client's attorney-in-fact or lawyer or from the lawyer of a client's attorney-in-fact.

On rare occasions, my client's adult child who's also the care giver has requested a CWA to inform a parent's future care. Usually, these assessments have been requested as a tool to deal with disagreements among family members. And some have been in response to a threat of guardianship proceedings.

With my reservations about comprehensive written assessments, why do I include so much detail in how to create one? Because, while you may not produce many in written form, *the assessment model that I lay out in the following chapter informs what you should keep in mind when working with clients and their families.* With or without a formal CWA, my model can frame your approach to a client and help you formulate recommendations. Starting with a review of CWAs will set the stage to understand all components of assessing your clients, written or not.

Chapter 11

Comprehensive Written Assessments

The *comprehensive written assessment* (CWA) is typically requested by a client's attorney-in-fact (AIF) or lawyer. My involvement may be limited to this assessment. CWAs may be used to resolve questions or disputes regarding a client's capacity to make his or her own medical and financial decisions and may determine the client's care needs.

I structure a CWA using specific categories. Generally, these are as follows:

Introduction

Why and by whom have I been asked to complete the assessment? If there is legal action involved, I state a specific reason for the request only if it has been provided by who requested the assessment.

In the introduction, I list who I interview (in addition to the client), and if relevant to the assessment, where the interviews occurred. Also, I list the reviewed reports and documents. Candidates for interviews include family members, care givers, physicians, and other professionals.

Examples of reports or documents might include a neurological evaluation, psychological assessment, and/or documentation of the most recent history and physical examination by the primary physician.

Though I have left them out in my examples, I include dates of interviews and exams.

* I'm asked to complete an assessment of Conrad J. by his lawyer, Alex. I interview Conrad and his daughter, Francine, at his home in Seattle. I speak with the two of them, tour the home with Conrad, and speak to Conrad privately. I talk to Conrad's primary physician and with her nurse. I also speak to Dr. L (internal medicine and nephrology), who is monitoring Conrad's kidney function. Francine provides a copy of the medical and psychological report by Elana B, PhD, for my review.

Checklist, introduction

- Name of the client
- Name of the person requesting the assessment
- Where the client was interviewed
- Names of those interviewed with the client
- Names of others interviewed and their relationship to the client
- Reports reviewed
- Documents reviewed

Presenting Issues

What is the reason for the assessment? Possibilities include (1) disagreement among family members as to the care needed, (2) dispute regarding cost and/or location of where and by whom the care is to be provided, and (3) guardianship proceedings are being considered or have been initiated.

You may be asked to compare estimated costs for recommended home care versus costs in an assisted care setting.

If the reason for the assessment is my client's current status (see below), I combine this section with the current status section.

* Conrad's four offspring disagree about his ability to make decisions regarding his care and finances. Conrad's eldest daughter, Leslie, filed a vulnerable adult petition[1] in the fall of last year and followed with a petition for guardianship, which was dismissed. In the spring of this year, Leslie files a second petition for guardianship.

Checklist, presenting issues

The following might be separate or combined under current status:

- The issue that initiated the request for the assessment
- Those involved in the issue

Psychosocial History

Information I record:

- Basic history: date and place of birth; where raised, current residence and how long lived there; cultural heritage, religious affiliation or belief system; sexual orientation
- Family: parents, siblings, and other family members. Does my client have siblings who are currently part of their lives or support system? Are there surviving siblings? Is there a troubled family history that affects their current relationships?
- Education, work, social, and marital history

Are there children and/or step-children, and/or grandchildren from a marriage, or marriages? If so, what are the children's and grandchildren's ages and places of residence? Do they live near my client?

[1]The Vulnerable Adult Petition is a law in some states that protects older adults.

Is my client's religion or faith relevant to his history and/or current situation? For example, did my client practice faith throughout his life and did that change as a result of current circumstances? Was my client raised in a religious family, yet severed ties with his faith background in adulthood?

I list groups or affiliations that have been and continue to be important to my client. I note any recent loss of a family member or close friend.

The following section provides the psychosocial information of the client's family of origin, significant adult relationships, social and work history, and where living family members and friends reside.

How the above affects the client is discussed later.

* Conrad was born on January 18, 1925, and was raised in Seattle, Washington, where he met Maxine. Conrad, five years older than Maxine, joined the service and moved to Montana. After graduating from high school, Maxine followed Conrad to Montana and they married. The couple later returned to Seattle where they raised a family. Conrad and Maxine had four children: a daughter, Leslie, a son, Victor (the eldest), a son, Perry, and a daughter, Francine (the youngest). In 1963, the family moved into the home where Conrad continues to live. Conrad and Maxine had been married 58 years when she died, eight years ago.

Throughout his adult life, Conrad has been active in the American Legion. He attends monthly meetings and goes to lunch regularly with friends he's made there. A week before my visit, one of these close friends died unexpectedly.

Checklist, psychosocial history

Information I record:

- Date and place of birth
- Parents and siblings
- Educational history

- Marital history, children and grandchildren
- Social history, including groups or affiliations
- Religious or faith history
- Recent losses of family members or friends

Current Status

This includes both objective and subjective impressions from meeting with the client. How does the client present himself? Is he meticulously, casually, or poorly groomed? In conversation, is he oriented to person, place, and time? Does he demonstrate confusion about his situation or about why you are interviewing him? Is he able to easily answer your questions or does he become confused, agitated, or tangential[2] in his responses? Is his facial expression (affect) appropriate to the conversation?

I record the client's living situation. Where does my client live; alone or with others?

I document the client's support system: family and paid care givers; support from neighbors, friends, faith group, clubs, and other affiliations.

(Note: The point of an assessment is usually for legal reasons, so I stick with the expected medical-model terms, such as "presents," i.e., what I observe of my client, in person, and "affect," i.e., my client's emotional expression, or lack there of.)

✻ Conrad presents as well-groomed, pleasant, and cooperative. His affect is open and engaged, although at times he appears confused. He looks to his daughter, Francine, to answer questions about dates, medical history, medications, and his current kidney dysfunction. When I ask about the guardianship proceedings, he does not understand the proceedings or why his children are in conflict about his care.

---

[2]Does he go off on verbal tangents?

Two of Conrad's adult children, Francine and Perry, live with him. Perry was already living in an apartment in the home, when in 1997, Francine moved in at her parents' request to assist them with household management and transportation. Francine prepares all meals for herself and her father, and Perry joins them for dinners. Francine does the shopping, cleaning, and laundry. She coordinates and accompanies Conrad to medical appointments, obtains and administers prescribed medications, and follows up on doctors' recommendations. Once a week, Conrad and Francine shop for groceries and go out to lunch.

Checklist, current status

- Is affect appropriate?
- Grooming
- Oriented to person, place, and time?
- Confusion, agitation, hostility, anger, defensiveness, tangentiality, confabulation
- Does client live alone? I note others who live with the client.
- Care system: care received from others, both paid and unpaid
- Support system: contact with family, friends, neighbors, groups, or clubs

Medical History

This category includes all relevant medical history and issues that led to my client's current medical care. Examples: a car accident that resulted in impaired mobility or cognition, or chronic pain; a disease from childhood, such as polio or childhood diabetes; vision or hearing loss; a history of a stroke, cancer, neurological disorder, or brain damage; a history of hospitalizations and surgeries, relevant to the current medical status; specialists being seen for chronic conditions; a history of falls; a history of depression, mental disorder, alcohol or drug abuse; if the client suffers from dementia, the date of diagnosis by the primary physician, and if available, testing done to reach the diagnosis.

* Conrad has a history of kidney disease and had surgery to remove his left kidney a year and a half ago. He also has a history of hypertension and hypothyroidism.

Checklist, medical history

- Chronic conditions, and history of treatment and/or surgery and hospitalizations
- History of depression or mental illness
- History of alcohol or drug abuse
- History of cancer, diabetes, heart disease, stroke, and treatment
- History of neurological disorder, such as Parkinson's Disease or multiple sclerosis
- History of childhood illness or impairments that continue to be treated and/or impair current functioning
- History of accidents that resulted in injuries that impair functioning
- History of falls

Medical Status

This section includes all current diagnoses and prescribed medications and/or treatment. This information is typically obtained from the most recent history and physical exam done by the client's primary physician or from the client or family care giver/advocate.

* Conrad is diagnosed with kidney disease, hypothyroidism, hypertension, gout, back pain, and Vitamin D and potassium deficiencies.

(I would include Conrad's complete medication list.)

Based on the testing of his kidney function, Conrad's primary physician refers him to nephrologist, Dr. L. Following additional testing, Dr. L recommends that Conrad attend classes about dialysis, as this is likely a consideration in his future.

Checklist, medical status

- All current diagnoses
- All current prescribed medications, treatment, and recommended treatment

Mental Status

This is a description of the client's cognitive status. If the client suffers from dementia, I note the level of impairment. I state if I advise 24-hour care and supervision.

If the primary physician has not diagnosed dementia, but family members have observed memory problems, I report that. Also, I report obvious impairment observed during my interview. If the client has recently been screened for dementia, I provide results.

I include signs of depression or mental disorder, such as hopelessness, anxiety, paranoia, and/or hallucinations.

* Conrad seems confused about the guardianship petition that has been filed by his eldest daughter, and he can't recall what medications he's on. However, he accurately recalls his high blood pressure and responds to Francine bringing up his kidney problems by stating he hopes he doesn't have to go on dialysis.

Francine reports that in recent months, she has noticed her father's memory worsening. On a mini-mental status exam (MMSE) given last fall, Conrad scored 30 of 30, indicating no cognitive impairment. On an MMSE given in May, Conrad scored 21 of 30, suggesting mild cognitive impairment. A screening tool indicated no present depression.

The MMSE is a screening device rather than a diagnostic tool; it's used to support a need for additional testing. Conrad's recent MMSE score of 21 of 30 is as yet unexplained. At this point, Conrad has not been diagnosed with dementia by his primary physician.

The report by Elana B, PhD, of April 12 (just before Conrad's most recent visit to his primary physician), states: "Conrad suffers from dementia that is progressing from mild to moderate," and "his condition is permanent and progressive."

I document that Conrad's cognitive impairment began when the family clashed over the management of Conrad's finances and care.

Checklist, mental status

- Diagnosis of dementia
- Memory impairment perceived during interview
- Depression, history of and/or current
- Mental disorder, history of and/or current
- Unusual behavior, such as paranoia, or delusions, such as talking to someone not present
- History of drug or alcohol abuse, and/or any present indications

Functional Status

This section includes a report of my client's ability, with or without assistance, to get around in and outside the home. I report where and how any falls have occurred. I note Adaptive Daily Living Skills (ADLS). I include personal care and household tasks, medications taken, meal preparation, shopping, scheduling of appointments, and transportation.

If they no longer have the skills to prepare balanced meals and drink sufficient fluids, my client's nutrition and hydration may be of concern. I include incontinence of bowel or bladder and how my client manages it. I report any type of assistance my client receives and from whom.

I discuss management of finances, including bill paying and tax preparation, and if my client has been a victim of phone, mail, or email fraud.

I report activities or behaviors that result in increased risk that are due to physical or mental difficulties: performing risky home maintenance tasks, such as cleaning gutters; wandering from their home and getting lost; car accidents; cooking accidents; or fires.

* Conrad is independent in all personal care—dressing, bathing, and grooming. He is continent of bowel and bladder. He walks without the use of assistive devices. He no longer drives.

As noted earlier, Conrad's daughter, Francine, manages his medications, prepares his meals, assists with errands, shopping, and laundry, and does much of the housekeeping.

Conrad remains socially active with friends and family. He enjoys television and has several favorite programs. He enjoys reading science fiction.

Checklist, functional status

- Mobility, including use of assistive devices: cane, walker, wheelchair, home adaptation
- Home environment, specific to safety concerns
- Assistance needed with adaptive daily living skills, and who provides the assistance
- Nutrition and hydration
- At-risk issues, due to impaired physical and/or cognitive function: use of stairs; wandering; resistance to care; poor hygiene or nutrition; accidents while driving; performing unsafe chores

Optional Sections

In some situations, I adjust the assessment to my client's circumstances. With Conrad, it's important to include the care provided by his offspring, so I add family care and client's expressed wishes.

Under family care, I detail the assistance Francine provides in the home, and that Francine and Victor contribute to home adaption, medical oversight and bill paying. I reference a long-term care policy Conrad had purchased. I also discuss the ongoing involvement of each of Conrad's offspring, such as visits and phone contact.

Client's Expressed Wishes

Given the guardianship petition, it's important to establish Conrad's wishes regarding his current and future care. I question Conrad privately; his responses are thoughtful and demonstrate good judgement.

* Conrad states that he would like to remain in his home as long as possible. He enjoys the company of Francine and Perry and would like them to continue living with him as long as they wish, stating, "We all get along pretty well." He understands that in the future, it may be necessary for him to live with other adults in an assisted care setting.

Recommendations

In this section, I include recommendations to be implemented immediately and in the future. Immediate recommendations are obvious: prevent an imminent risk to my client's health and/or safety. For example, I may recommend a home safety evaluation and assessment that includes the possible need for adaptive equipment. Risks include the possibility of leaving a burning pot on the stove, the risk of a fall when climbing steep stairs or when bathing, or having to negotiate a cluttered environment.

If cognitive impairment or possible depression is reported or noted, I might request an evaluation from the primary physician.

This is also the section where I recommend any future involvement as care consultant or manager.

* **Recommendations Itemized:**

- Further medical and psychological testing to ascertain if Conrad's recent cognitive decline indicates dementia.
- Francine and Victor continue to oversee finances and medical care.
- For future homecare needs, review Conrad's long-term care policy.
- Consider care consultation for Conrad's adult children; help them come to an agreement to provide the support that Conrad needs for future health challenges.
- Consider care management for ongoing assessment of Conrad's needs to help with set up of future services.

Checklist, recommendations

- Recommendations about urgent and long-term care
- Urgent risks, such as falling
- Needs of attention, such as hygiene, nutrition, medication management, transportation
- Recommendations of further testing
- Client's wishes regarding future care
- Cost of future care

Chapter 12

Care Assessment of Josephine B.

I'm asked to complete an assessment of Josephine (Josie) by her daughter, Angie, and son, Lance, who are Josie's co-attorneys-in-fact (AIF). The assessment is requested because Lance has concerns about the care provided by the adult family home, Golden Views, where Josie resides. Lance is especially concerned about the amount of stimulation provided at Golden Views. Lance has explored dementia care options for Josie and has taken Josie to visit facilities. He also wonders whether it's feasible for Josie to return to her own home. Angie, on the other hand, is satisfied with their mother's current care.

I meet separately with Josie, Angie, and Lance. I interview Lillian S, RN, owner and operator of Golden Views adult family home, where Josie resides.

I review the adult family home assessment, the negotiated care plan, their chart notes, and a report on the neuro-behavioral status exam performed by Carolyn R, RN, PhD (nursing) on Josie four months after her admittance to Golden Views. I also speak with Shauna, Josie's private companion and care giver.

Psychosocial History

Josie was born on January 6, 1931, in Pittsburgh, Pennsylvania. She married Robert in 1958. Soon after getting married, Josie and Robert went to live in India for two years. Josie took photos of the people, wildlife, and scenery.

Josie and Robert returned from India to settle in California. They had two children, a daughter, Angie, and a son, Lance.

Josie, who attributes her time in India with stimulating her interest in anthropology, earned her master's degree in anthropology from UCLA. She went on to teach animal behavior to middle-school students in California. Her son, Lance, remembers that she enjoyed teaching and was loved by her students and fellow teachers.

After 38 years of marriage, Josie divorced her husband. Following, she purchased a 35-acre farm in a rural area and moved there 12 years ago. Four years later, Josie's daughter Angie and Angie's family moved to a home nearby.

Lance lives in Montana and visits his mother regularly. Josie reports that her ex-husband, with whom she continues to be on good terms, also visits her on occasion.

Medical Status

A year and a half ago, Josie was living in her home on the farm and fell while walking down the stairs. She sustained a fracture of her right tibia and was hospitalized and treated. For rehabilitation, she was transferred to a skilled nursing facility. Eleven days later, she was hospitalized and treated for a fractured neck, also a consequence of the original fall. At discharge from the hospital, Josie was placed at Golden Views Adult Family Home.

Current diagnoses include irritable bowel syndrome, osteoporosis, Alzheimer's disease, and depression.

Medications include Citalopram, 30mg daily for depression; Aricept 10mg daily and Namenda 5mg daily for memory loss; Boniva, 1 tab monthly for osteoporosis; and pseudoephedrine as needed for allergies. In addition, Josie takes vitamins.

Her irritable bowel syndrome causes frequent diarrhea that results in anal irritation, which is treated with nystatin ointment and sitz baths. Due to the colitis, Josie's diet is carefully monitored.

Josie suffers constant pain from her neck fracture. The pain is managed by steroid injections from her primary physician, with Tylenol added as needed.

Cognitive Status

Josie was diagnosed with Alzheimer's disease five years ago by her primary physician. In my conversation with Josie, I observe that she has difficulty with word finding and is tangential when responding to questions.

Four months after admission to Golden Views, Carolyn R, RN, PhD, administered a neurobehavioral cognitive status examination. Josie was found to be moderately impaired in judgement and severely impaired in memory and orientation. According to adult family home operator, Lillian S, Josie's impairments cause her to be unaware of her limitations and put her at risk for falls and wandering. On one occasion, Josie had to be redirected when heading out the gate of Golden Views. On other occasions, Josie insists that she wants to walk to the home of her daughter, Angie, in order to help her.

Josie was diagnosed with depression seven years ago by her primary physician. Angie suspects the onset of her mother's depression followed her divorce.

Current Status and Presenting Issues

Josie has resided at Golden Views for a year and eight months. There are four other adults being cared for in the home. Josie eats meals in the dining room with the other residents. She participates in all activities, including holiday and birthday celebrations. Josie enjoys working in the garden and especially likes to water the organic patch.

Josie's private care giver, Shauna, takes her shopping, to appointments with doctors (often accompanied by Angie), and to visit Josie's own home. In addition to appointments, Shauna's scheduled time is Monday and Thursday, from 1 to 5 p.m. Shauna reports that during their times together, Josie says she is ready to go home, or wants to go home (to her farm).

Josie also frequently visits Angie and her husband, Trent, and their five-year-old son, Will.

During my meeting with Josie, she's confused about the plan for her future. Despite my assurances that she and her children will discuss her future care, Josie asks if I'm going to place her in a facility. She states, "I will be going home soon" (to her farm). In a later conversation, Josie says, "I'm not sure I want to live on the farm," and shortly, thereafter, "I think I want to keep the farm and continue to visit."

Josie recalls that "we did a lot of looking at places to live," and though she thinks they're all "wonderful," she prefers "to be on my own and going places." When asked what she thinks her children want for her, she's aware they disagree. Josie also states that she wants to see Angie and Lance as much as possible. She expresses deep affection for her grandson, Will, and says she enjoys the time she spends with him.

Following my interview with Josie, Lance informs me that he no longer feels that a dementia care facility is appropriate. Lance asked me to provide an estimate for home care.

Estimated Cost of Home Care

Because she suffers from Alzheimer's disease, Josie requires 24/7 supervision. She also requires nursing oversight to address her irritable bowel syndrome. Josie requires careful dietary management and treatment of frequent diarrhea. My report includes two options for the required home care.

I speak with Beth, RN, the owner/operator of a homecare agency that provides service to the area. Their live-in rate is $325 per day. However, because of the need for nurse delegation of the prescription ointment used to treat anal irritation, state guidelines require that the hourly rate is charged, rather than a live-in rate. The cost would jump to $612 per day or approximately $18,360 per month. In addition, nurse care management would range from $3800 to $4400 the first month, and approximately $1425 to $1800 per month thereafter.

I also speak with a nurse care manager, Doreen K of DLK Care Consultation. As a private geriatric nurse care manager, Doreen hires and supervises care givers who she places in the home and can delegate tasks to the care givers without being subject to state requirements. Doreen quotes a daily rate for live-in care of $380 per day or approximately $11,400 per month.

Because the farm is in a remote area, Doreen would have to recruit and hire care givers to provide the live-in care, which would increase the costs. The charge for setting up the services would be approximately $2500 for the first month. Doreen estimates that the care management costs for the first month would exceed $3250 (which is in addition to the live-in care). Doreen also estimates that ongoing charges for nurse care management would be higher due to the remote location and would be approximately $2175 per month. I did not discuss with Doreen whether travel time would be charged for the live-in care givers.

The minimum cost for live-in care and nurse care management adds up to $13,575 per month. This rate reflects live-in care givers, who are also expected to clean the home, purchase groceries and supplies, cook meals, and do the laundry. The quoted amount does not reflect the cost for groceries and supplies, increased utility expenses, and so on. As Josie's dementia increases, the cost of care is likely to increase, considerably. Because Josie is at high risk for falls, and in the future, wandering, additional services, such as housekeeping, shopping, and meal preparation may have to be added to free the care givers to attend to Josie. If Josie requires awake care at night, this would further increase the cost.

Summary and Recommendations

Josie is receiving needed care at Golden Views adult family home. She has a lovely private room in a large home, with beautiful grounds. The home is amply staffed, and there are four other elders for Josie to socialize with. Three times a week, accompanied by her private care giver, Shauna, she is able to visit her home on the farm. She visits with her daughter and family one to four times a week, and Angie calls Josie frequently.

From my discussions with Josie, it's clear she's confused by the possibility for a change of residence. She is further confused by the conflicting opinions between Angie and Lance. In my discussions with Josie, and with other involved parties, Josie is ambivalent, at best, about a return to live in her own home.

My recommendations:

- Because Josie suffers from Alzheimer's disease, she's incapable to decide where she receives care. That's the responsibility of her attorneys-in-fact, Angie and Lance.

- Angie and Lance should reach a decision as soon as possible whether Josie will continue at Golden Views or if she will move to her home and receive home care. I recommend Josie stay at Golden Views.
- To assure Josie they're in agreement, Angie and Lance should meet with Josie to convey their decision.
- If Angie and Lance agree that Josie remain at Golden Views, to address Lance's concerns, I recommend facilitated conversations between Lance and Golden Views operator, Lillian S.
- If she remains at Golden Views, Josie's visits to her farm home, accompanied by Shauna, should continue, with careful attention to Josie's safety. Josie's level of fatigue, and other behavior or response when returning to Golden Views, should be monitored.
- Angie and Lance should assemble a simple photo album with a captioned history of Josie's life. The album should include photos of recent activities with family and photos of her care team. As dementia progresses, the album will be a helpful tool.
- If Angie and Lance decide that Josie will return to her home, a home safety evaluation should be completed. This can be arranged by the hired nurse care manager.
- Finally, I recommend that, before the meeting in which they convey their decision to their mother, Angie, Lance, and I meet to discuss this report to make sure they're in agreement.

Chapter 13

Care Assessment of Gary Bloom

The following care assessments of Gary Bloom and Joan McGinnis are fictitious—as this is written, it takes place in the future—and is based partially on facts and partially on non-facts. We did this exercise to encourage all who plan to enter this profession to do their own future care assessment. Envisioning your future care assessment can deepen empathy for your clients.

The text within brackets are observations that aren't included in the written assessment.

September 1, 2026

Gary Bloom and his wife, Joan (who made the initial contact), request an assessment of Gary. I meet with the couple in my office, initially, and in their home, a week later.

Psychosocial History

Gary was born in Chicago, in 1948, grew up in Los Angeles, and spent his adult years in the Bay Area and Seattle area. He married Joan in 1984, the first and only marriage for both. They had a son in 1986, who lives in Seattle, and a daughter in 1990, who lives in Portland. Gary was a licensed marriage and family counselor, with a career in the mental health field. He currently writes nonfiction. Joan was a social worker. Gary and Joan live in a two-story home in Edmonds.

Both adult children are on good terms with Gary and Joan, and they visit regularly.

> [From our meeting and this brief history, I'm able to make several assumptions. First, that the family does not have significant conflicts, which will make agreements smoother. Second, that Gary's cognitive abilities appear to be largely intact.]

Medical Status

Gary has a tendency to high blood pressure, which he manages with diet and exercise.

Gary suffers from neuropathy in primarily his right foot and occasionally in his left foot. His symptoms are most present after a long walk, lifting something heavy, or sitting in a conventional chair for long periods. He also suffers from back stiffness after sitting for a long time, especially when he must use a conventional chair instead of his ergonomic chair at home. His symptoms first appeared in 2012, following what he deems overuse or poor form on a rowing machine. Following the injury, he was treated by a physical therapist, which helped alleviate the pain.

Gary reports that he has mild short-term memory loss—forgetting names of acquaintances, occasionally, and some problems with recalling words. On the other hand, he reports that he can still put together a complex essay and is even trying to create a simple video game.

Gary still works out regularly and practices (with Joan) Tai Chi most mornings. Along with his back issues, he suffers from chronic tendinitis in his left elbow. Every couple of years, he sustains a new injury, typically from overdoing a workout. He usually forgoes seeing his doctor, instead choosing treatments from his physical therapist (PT) that typically last several months. His explanation is that his PT does a better job of diagnosing injuries, and "doctors don't offer any treatment, anyway."

Gary is not on any medications. He takes two ibuprofen about once a month, mostly due to back pain.

Cognitive Status

Aside from the minor short-term memory issues, neither Gary nor Joan see signs of Gary suffering from cognitive impairment. He solves his short-term memory problems by recording on his smart phone, tasks, notes, or ideas he needs to remember.

> [I have gathered that Gary won't concede his decisions to experts (me, in this case) or family members; he'll make his own decisions. How did I figure this? Because he states he chooses his own health treatments, and the authority in how he said that. Hence, the way to work with him will be to present facts and options, and suggest that he discuss them with his wife and choose among his (and their) options.
>
> An additional clue that Gary will take charge of his own treatment is that he chooses his PT over his doctor to treat injuries. At the same time, I observe that he respects his wife's opinions and is sensitive to her concerns. Any recommendations I make should be addressed to her as well as to him.]

Current Status and Presenting Issues

Gary lives with Joan in a two-story home in Edmonds, about 12 miles north of Seattle. With his off-and-on injuries, he considers the house and yard too much to maintain, both in cleaning and repair. He would like to sell the house and move to a small home with a small yard.

He and Joan are in conflict regarding the house. While the house is of modest size (1650 square feet), the lot is a quarter acre, on which Joan has created a complex garden that surrounds the lawn. Since Joan's retirement, five years ago, the garden has been the center of her life.

While generally in good health, Joan also suffers from some physical maladies, specifically arthritis, mostly in her hands. She is less able to tend to the garden on her own. Rather than move, Joan wishes to hire help, both for inside the home for cleaning and for help in the yard.

Gary hates the idea of spending money that he'd like to save for their children's inheritance and Joan's future care (Gary expects to die many years before his wife); and he believes that they should spend more time helping with the grandchildren than with taking care of a household.

Last, while Gary dislikes complex cooking and Joan enjoys it, Gary does the bulk of the cooking half the year because Joan is busy in the garden until the evening.

If Gary had his way, he would spend most of his time, reading, writing and pursuing other creative activities, and engaging in his exercise program.

> [Gary wishes to make concessions to their age-related infirmities and situation by downsizing. Joan's life is tied up in experimenting with sustainable gardening and feels that she has too much invested—in time, labor, and most of all, sentiment—in her yard of 40-plus years.
>
> While the couple appear to love and support each other, this issue has driven them into ongoing conflict for many

months. They admit that they are unable to discuss the issue, as neither can envision a compromise. They no longer even try to discuss it.

The concern is that they will avoid seeking any possible resolution. This could lead to increased marital conflict and create the possibility that nothing will change until a crisis (perhaps a major injury) presents itself.]

Estimated Cost of Household and Yard Help

The possibility of a compromise rests on providing services to assist with the yard and household chores. House cleaning service costs around $150 per 4-hour visit from an agency, but $100 to $120 for a private cleaner. Twice a month, split the difference, and say $220 per month for house cleaning. Joan estimates that she could make do with six hours a month help in her yard. At $30 an hour, that comes to $180. In the Pacific Northwest, yard and gardening work is a focus for about seven months a year. I'm rounding the yearly cost to about $4000, annually, for household and yard help, about $333 per month.

I also price some easy-to-prepare food at Costco and some other places, and it would cost very little more for Joan and Gary to eat easy-to-prepare meals a couple days a week.

Last, Gary and Joan have both expressed interest in helping their daughter with child care, which would require spending extended time in Portland. I look at the home and apartment rental prices in Portland and for how much they could rent their Edmonds residence. They would be looking at somewhere between a $500 and $1000 profit in that exchange.

[I don't know how Gary and Joan will feel about spending $4000 a year on house and garden assistance, but we will at least have a concrete choice for them to consider. They could also compromise: they could have the house cleaned once a month instead of twice. Joan could exchange some of her maintenance-intensive vegetation with some plants and bushes that take less work.]

Summary and Recommendations

While Gary is in good health and condition, he is finding it increasingly discomforting to do some housework he has always done and even finds some meal preparation he does beyond his comfort level. While their home is modest by current standards, there is still much to take care of and more room than necessary for a couple. Gary and Joan have never had household help, and Joan only occasionally hires help for her yard work. Gary wishes to explore a move to a smaller (more manageable) home and yard, while Joan is insistent in not leaving her beloved yard.

> [While Gary would be making the biggest compromise, by agreeing to remain in their current home, his concern for Joan would likely mean he would cooperate if his household responsibilities were lessened. As far as moving temporarily to Portland, Joan would have to make that decision.]

I recommend that

- Because Gary is becoming less capable of some of his household chores and wishes to focus his physical activity on what makes him feel physically better, I suggest they start with hiring a household cleaner to come in once per month. As neither Gary nor Joan are neatness fanatics, once a month may be sufficient to augment any household cleaning the couple wishes to continue themselves.

- Because of their mutual concern for Joan's physical well-being, I recommend that she hire yard help for three hours a month, seven months a year.
- Because Gary is uncomfortable with preparing complex meals, I recommend that they engage a prepared meal service, starting with one per week. Joan should also agree to expect Gary to prepare mostly easy-to-make meals (such as salmon burgers).
- They should explore with each other and their daughter how it would work for Gary and Joan to move to Portland temporarily. However, because of Joan's reluctance to leave her yard for extended periods, they could do an experiment—keep their house and visit Portland for extended stays.

Chapter 14

Care Assessment of Joan Bloom

The text within brackets are observations that aren't included in the written assessment.

September 1, 2026

I'm asked to do a care assessment of Joan Bloom, at her request, to assist in planning for current and potential future care for Joan and her husband, Gary. I first meet Joan in my office, then visit the couple in their home. For this assessment, I did not contact Joan's physician, as the necessary medical information was obtained from Joan.

Psychosocial History

Joan was born in 1951, in New Castle, Pennsylvania. She was the youngest child and only daughter of loving parents from very different backgrounds and temperaments. She grew up with a half-brother from her mother's first marriage, 12 years older (and since deceased), and with a brother, two years older.

Joan's mother was born in Wales to an English father and mother. She moved to the States when she was 11 years old. Joan affectionately describes her father's family as "country bumpkins." Joan recalls her grandfather, father, and uncles playing bluegrass music at family get-togethers.

Joan, a social worker, attributes her early interest in the field to her parents' contrasting temperaments and communication styles. She earned a master's degree in social work and worked in the field until her retirement at age 70.

Joan and Gary married in 1984, had a son in 1986, and a daughter in 1990. They have lived in the same two-story home, with a quarter-acre lot, since 1989. Their son lives in Seattle and their daughter lives in Portland, Oregon. Joan is close to both her children and views them as part of the couples' support system. Joan is also close to her surviving brother, who lives in the Bay Area.

Medical Status

Joan has osteoarthritis, primarily in her hands. Her right hand has noticeable swelling in the joints of her index and middle fingers. In addition to being moderately painful, it affects her manual dexterity and interferes with her favorite pastime, gardening, and at times with cooking. Joan has a large organic garden in which she grows many fruits, vegetables, herbs, and flowers. The benefactors of her garden include family, friends and "the critters." She also likes to make jam, pesto, and meals, from her produce—activities that entail harvesting, cleaning and chopping. Joan does hand exercises to decrease her joint stiffness.

The osteoarthritis also affects her knees, primarily, when she climbs the stairs in her home and when she dances to her favorite rock music.

Joan suffers from tinnitus in her left ear, which has resulted in slight hearing loss. The possibility of a tumor (a possible cause of tinnitus when in only one ear) has been ruled out. Joan has adjusted to the constant ringing and becomes concerned only when the sound intensifies or also occurs in her right ear. As these episodes are becoming more frequent, she worries that someday the increased ringing will become constant.

Joan's grandmother had glaucoma and was prescribed daily eye drops. Her mother was diagnosed with narrow-angle glaucoma, with a risk of eye pressure spiking. Because of this genetic history, Joan receives regular eye exams.

Joan takes no medications, other than occasional ibuprofen for arthritis-related pain.

Cognitive Status

Although neither Joan nor Gary have noticed significant problems with her memory, Joan's biggest fear is that she will eventually succumb to Alzheimer's disease. Joan's mother, who died 12 days before her 96th birthday, was diagnosed with Alzheimer's disease when she was in her early 80s. Her mother also had osteoarthritis with the telltale swollen joints of her hands, and tinnitus. While Joan is far more dedicated than her mother in health habits—diet, and exercise of body and mind—Joan remains concerned.

Current Status and Presenting Issues

In the years Joan and Gary have lived in their current home, their large yard has become Joan's palette to pursue her passion for gardening, and eventually, an interest in permaculture. When she retired as a social worker, five years ago, this interest became her life's purpose. As Joan describes it: "My husband's passion is what he reads, thinks, and writes about. My passion is in my relationships with people, nature, and its many creatures. My husband can do what he loves anywhere. I need a yard to do what I love and share with others."

This difference in interests, and context for exploring them, has led to their main disagreements in how their aging together will unfold. Gary evaluates cost to maintain their home, indoors and outdoors. He would prefer to downsize to a smaller home. He's concerned about the limitation that Joan's arthritis imposes on her ability to maintain her garden and the potential for injury that he could sustain if he assisted. In contrast, Joan views her home and garden as a creative outlet, part of her exercise habits, and an environment to entertain and share with family and friends.

Joan concedes that many gardening tasks have become difficult, such as pruning the fruit and ornamental trees and bushes. She has designed her garden so that most beds are covered with vegetation, but weeding continues to be needed and the grass must be mowed.

Joan and Gary have no interest in moving to a retirement/assisted living facility.

> [During a tour of Joan's garden, it's clear how much value she places on the garden for cognitive stimulation and for her need for community. Joan describes Sunday "food shares" that she sponsors in her yard during the summer, when neighbors and friends can come to share in the bounty of her garden and trade offerings of their own. Given how strongly Joan feels about her need to retain her palette for her current passion, I assume selling their home is not up for discussion. While neither Joan nor Gary are passive, go-along types, they take each other's needs seriously and will have to work out their differences over time. My recommendations will focus on aging in their present home but can be applied to wherever they choose to live.]

Summary and Recommendations

The couple's disagreement about remaining in their current home or downsizing to a smaller, more manageable home is theirs to resolve. My recommendations will focus on aging in their present home, but can apply to wherever they choose to live. I considered three issues:

- Yard work: Increase number of low-maintenance plants in the yard. Hire a service that will prune trees and bushes. As the couple is adept at using the Internet, I don't recommend particular businesses to do this work. I estimate the initial cost could exceed $1000. Every other year, continue to maintain the trees and bushes. The cost should be considerably less once the initial work is done. Joan spoke of friendly relations with several neighborhood teenagers. I recommend hiring one or two of them to mow the lawn, weed, and possibly, harvest.
- Home adaptation: Although not currently needed, the couple should be prepared to adapt their home in case of increased physical impairment and to reduce their risk of falls. Given that falls often occur when bathing and when climbing stairs, I suggest they consider these changes: A ramp to their front porch, which is two steps up; turn their den on the main floor into a master bedroom, with a walk-in tub in the laundry area, which would eliminate the need to regularly use the stairs to the second floor and provide maximum safety in bathing.
- If they decide to move to a smaller home, eventually, be sure that the home is one story, level entry, and can be adapted for wheelchair use and safe bathing. Also, evaluate a potential new yard in terms of accessibility and required maintenance and the associated costs.

Part IV

Working with Families

Chapter 15

The Accidental Care Giver

You may have heard this before: Put a frog in a pot of water and set the burner to simmer. If the change in temperature is sufficiently gradual, by the time the frog experiences pain, it will be too late to escape. (Please don't try this at home.)

Could you be that frog? It starts simply. While shopping, you pick up a few items for your elderly, widowed father. As time goes on, you get more and more items for him and make extra stops at various stores. Before you know it, you've taken on all his shopping and errands. Next, the laundry becomes too difficult for Dad. So, being the dutiful daughter, you're now washing, drying, and folding his clothes. Dad begins to have difficulty cooking, so you bring over a couple of meals a week. Then, well, you get the picture. Before you know it, you're neglecting your own household and work responsibilities and are so stressed you're ready to implode.

And what does Dad think about your help? He thinks he needn't spend any money on his care because "my daughter takes care of it." He has learned to take your assistance for granted and so have you. Both of you forget how much you do and how long it takes to do it. If Dad has dementia, it's even worse; he may forget all the "little" things you handle.

While Dad is proud of his ability to live "independently," you, being human, are growing resentful of the increasing time you spend caring for him. So you bring up the possibility of hiring help and come up against his attitude towards money; i.e., he doesn't want to spend any. He may even play the guilt card to ensure that you continue to pick up all the chores he's no longer capable of handling. So there you are, boiling like the frog, and you can't jump out.

Here's another example of a care giver in a pot. Your wife, who suffers from multiple sclerosis, is experiencing a steady decline and is becoming dependent on you for all her care. She can no longer move from her wheelchair without help, so you must be with her all the time. Actually, someone must be with her, but she will accept help from no one but her husband. She is unwilling to recognize the amount of stress that results from providing constant aid, and you are unable to identify and state your needs. The situation moves to the breaking point when you are diagnosed with cancer and must undergo chemotherapy.

Getting That Call

On many occasions (perhaps the majority of them), I've gotten that call from an accidental care giver, a family member of an elder who can no longer fend for himself or herself and has gotten used to the family member sliding into the role as the care giver. And, likely, the caller will be frustrated with the elder, and perhaps with other family members, over who is doing what and who isn't. For these reasons among others, my first meeting with the family might be full of conflict.

Chapter 16

Introduction to Working With Families

Soon after Mom and Dad arrive home from the hospital with your new little sister or brother, rather than the puppy you were hoping for, you realize that siblings are a mixed bag. Your parents will start using the word "share" a lot, which means you'll be sharing resources you'd taken for granted as yours and yours alone—affection, attention, things money can buy.

Over time, multiple siblings leads to more than sharing, it leads to factions and alliances. Some of these factions and alliances change with the rate of the weather, while others change with the rate of pre-historic eras. Some include one or more parents. (I say more, not both, because of step-parents.) Some are factions of one. And these are not just childhood alliances, they stretch through lifetimes.

Don't look for alliances among siblings to make sense, especially when parents are included. Adult children that stay to help elderly parents may not be a favorite of those parents. One or more of the parents may identify with and favor the adventurous offspring that moved thousands of miles away[1] and visits every couple of years; or the flakey offspring might be favored over the responsible ones.[2] Throughout their lives, adult siblings can stay close in geography, relationships, or both, or go their own way in geography, relationships, or both. However, when decisions about their parents' care arise, the close friendships, or at least, treaties among adult siblings may dissolve into bickering.

As a care consultant, you will deal with siblings who disagree with each other on the care of their parents. When the family is willing, I deal with these conflicts through family sessions, which as I detail below, is different from family therapy. It's either these sessions or have family conflicts leak into conversations and decisions regarding my client, and obviously, not in a good way.

If you use the GPS-based Google or Apple Directions app, when you're about to hit a traffic slowdown, the warning on the dynamic map will be displayed as color changes in the road, a change to orange for slowed traffic and to red for bumper-to-bumper. And you'll get a suggestion to use, if available, an alternate route. Unfortunately (or not), neither Google nor Apple has yet made a *Directions app* for family sessions. If they did, there are several hazards that would turn a path red for the care consultant: (1) mistaking family sessions for family therapy (both you and the family), (2) confusion regarding who's your client, and (3) being so preoccupied with your own concerns for your client, you forget to attend to the concerns of the family members.

[1] This is depicted in the movie, *Home for the Holidays.*

[2] This is depicted in the movie, *Parenthood.*

Chapter 17

A Family Session Is Not Family Therapy

You and the elder's children are moving through the session smoothly, when what seems to come out of nowhere, one sibling lashes out at another. Ouch! Where did *that* come from? Unless you were one of the five people on Earth who grew up without a bit of resentment towards attention-hogging siblings and family pets (and those five people are lying), you know exactly where that came from. Family members, sitting in a room, discussing sensitive family related issues? It feels like therapy, and we all know that during therapy it's okay—expected—to reveal hidden and sometimes profound emotions. Family therapy and care-related family sessions have so much in common that both care consultants and their clientele often confuse one with the other. Care mediation suffers from the *if it looks and quacks like a duck, it must be a duck* syndrome. But a care-related family session is not family therapy.

First, the similarities between family therapy and a care-related family session. A care-related family session often includes family members of more than one generation, and nearly always, one or more siblings. Those present have been brought together to solve a problem that has become intractable. One or two of those present may be the focus of that problem. Most participants have a history, about which they have varying opinions and attitudes, and that history results in mixed emotions about each other. As mentioned above, there are often numerous alliances and conflicts among the members.

Now let's look at the differences between family therapy and a care-related family session. In the latter, the children are nearly always adults and are looking after the needs of their parents rather than the other way around. The client may not be present in the session.[1] The siblings don't live together, lessening their need to get along with each other. While there may be significant cross-generational issues, everyone is a grown-up and may do as they wish—although the client may be (legally declared) incapacitated to make certain decisions. Potential inheritance—money—is the tyrannosaurus rex in the room.

There's one additional difference, and for the care consultant, it's the one that counts. It's the one you have to remember when a participant first confuses these care meetings with family therapy and unloads both barrels on someone in the session—maybe a sibling, maybe a parent, maybe you. Experience tells you that, once the congeniality force-field gets lowered for even a moment, the dung will hit the wind-powered energy generator: those factions among siblings and elders will pop-up so fast, and in such number, that you'll need to launch the spreadsheet to keep count.

If you've kept your wits about you, this difference will whisper in your ear: *It's time to hit the pause button before you and the family fall down a rabbit-hole of such chaos that it would make Lewis Carroll renounce fantasy.*

---

[1]In family therapy, the therapist may work with children's issues by working with only the parents—but that's less common than leaving the elderly client out of a care-consultation family session.

You're going to have to jump through all stages of, "Oh, hell!"—from denial to acceptance—in moments, because the only person that pause button works on is you.

What you have to keep front and center is that family therapy and family sessions have different goals. While in family therapy, the "identified client" is nearly always a child who is misbehaving in some fashion—skipping school, disrupting classrooms, doing drugs, running away, and so on—the client is typically viewed by the family therapist as one who is "acting out" to take the heat off the real problem. For example, Johnny disrupts his school classes because as long as he's the problem his parents stop bickering and (in Johnny's mind) won't get a divorce. The family therapist understands that Johnny won't stop acting out until his parents' marital issues are dealt with. Whether the marital issues are dealt with directly or by way of Johnny's problems is based on the approach of the family therapist, but dealt with they must be if Johnny is going to change his behavior.

The goal of family therapy must include, because all these family members live together, the need to get along well enough for that to continue. And to make that happen, your job as a family therapist may be to help them change the complex family dynamics.

In contrast, the care consultant's job is to be concerned with the family dynamics in only how they immediately interfere with the goal of setting up and maintaining care for the client. All the work in the session should be to that end. This does not mean that the care consultant can ignore family dynamics or that a knowledge of family systems theory is unnecessary. It's important to know what influences are present during the negotiations among family members. A 40-year-old adult child's concerns may be as complex, indirect, and unconscious as is with the disruptive Johnny. However, as a care consultant, my interest is to minimize the focus on matters that are disruptive rather than constructive to our task of setting up care. I respectfully acknowledge feelings that have caused conflict, but I do not let them take over the session.

Chapter 18

Who's the Client?

In the mid-80s, Larry Bird was the most brazen and competitive player in the NBA. The Boston Celtics forward was so good, that to avoid boredom, he would find ways to challenge himself during games. The right-hander once handicapped himself by spending an entire half shooting with only his left hand.

If you want to be the Larry Bird of care consultants, you can challenge yourself by taking advantage of an opportunity at the beginning of a contact or in initial family sessions. Before we get to that, please read the following scenarios with the following question in mind: Who's the client?

The daughter of an elder contacts you. She gives this account: Her father is maintaining marginally at home. He attends a day program three days a week, but she feels this is not enough to provide the support that he needs. Her brother will be the attorney-in-fact (AIF), if and when the DPOA[1] is activated, but it has yet to be activated, since Dad is still capable of making his own decisions. However, because Dad has not dealt well with his finances and is now in debt, her brother

[1]The DPOA is the document that identifies the attorney-in-fact and his or her specific authority.

has stepped in to pay bills that Dad can't cover. Because her brother is paying the bills, he believes that he should make all the important decisions for their father, even to the extent of telling Dad not to take prescribed anti-depressants because he (her brother) believes them to be ineffective.

Who's the client? The daughter who hired you and signed your fee agreement? The son who's been appointed the AIF, is paying father's bills, and might even be expected by the daughter to pay for your services because, after all, you're going to be evaluating their father's needs and making recommendations? Let's look at a few additional examples.

A woman suffers from early Alzheimer's disease. Her daughter has arranged for home care, but those services are insufficient to address that her mother is no longer able to prepare meals or take prescribed medications without supervision. Her daughter manages her finances and knows that the needed 24-hour home care is too expensive. Her daughter contacts you because she wants you to talk to her mother—who still (legally) makes her own decisions—into moving to an assisted living facility.

Who's the client? The daughter who hired you? Or her mother who, while suffering from cognitive disabilities and memory loss, still has the legal right to make her own decisions?

Finally: You are hired by a lawyer, the AIF for an elderly woman, on whose behalf asks for your assistance in dealing with the assisted living facility where she resides. You contact the facility, and the director complains that the AIF's client is disruptive and that they've exhausted their repertoire in trying to deal with her. But, much to your pleasant surprise, the director gushes over your stellar reputation and states that she's delighted that you will solve their problems with this woman.

Who's the client? The lawyer who hired you? Or the gushing director of the facility?

Who's the Client for Dummies

In nearly all professions, determining who's your client is simple. If you're a doctor, your client (or patient) is the one with the booboo, and is always the one under whose name the service is charged. If you're a lawyer, your client is going to be the one for whom you'll be advocating or defending. If you're an accountant, your client will be the one whose financial interests you'll be looking out for. If you're a counselor—okay, that one can get a little tricky,[2] but it's clear that the care consultant deals with confusion about who's the client more than other professionals.

So how can you be the Larry Bird of care consultation? How can you handicap your work with your clients? By regarding anyone but the elder as your client. No matter what, in your practice, you're going to be dealing with conflicts among those involved with an elder in need. People have differences of opinion, and those differences will often be the reason you're hired. But it's one thing to work to resolve the conflicts among the elder's posse, it's another thing to be conflicted about who's the client. You don't want to spend your time trying to solve conflicts within yourself. Even Larry Bird avoided that challenge while doing his job.

When numerous parties are involved, and if there are conflicts, your work can get difficult. But if you're having an especially hard time, ask yourself: Did I forget who the client is?

How it Happens, How to Avoid It.

When you've been hired, you're being paid twice: you're being paid money (indirectly, if you work in an agency), and you're being paid

[2] If you're a family therapist, while there may be an *identified client* required for insurance reimbursement, a family or marriage counselor might view the collective group as the client.

a professional compliment. It's normal to feel gratitude towards the person who made the decision to retain your services, and it goes against one's inclination to respond with *thank you for hiring me, but don't expect to be favored over the other parties.*

Nevertheless, you can get that across by making it clear that the elder is your client, and that every involved party is important in how they can serve the goal of assisting you in coming up with a plan and executing that plan to serve the needs of the client.

Getting across that the elder is the (one and only) client takes persistence. It will be reflected in how you gather information in that, unless demonstrated otherwise, no family member will be considered a more reliable informant than any other. It will be reflected in the manner of sharing information among those involved. I make it clear that I will share information as necessary, and only as necessary, in how it helps me create a care plan for the elder. It will be reflected, most of all, in the care plan itself.

At the same time, focusing on the needs of the client does not mean ignoring the needs of everyone else. To continue to give the best care, even parents of a newborn need to eat, sleep, and relax. That goes for all who assist in the care (whether directly or indirectly) of the elderly client. If a member of the family is taking on the bulk of responsibility by taking the client to appointments, paying her bills, or acting as a care giver, providing relief for that person is in the best interest of your client.

Are There Exceptions?

In sixteen years of private practice,[3] on two occasions, I was hired when the elder would not be involved, would not be my client.[4] The family

[3] as of this book's publication date

[4] I suppose this is where I say, "it's the exception that proves the rule," but I've never figured out what that means.

member needed advice on dealing with someone who would be unwilling to be my client. In both cases, my service took only a few hours. The takeaway is, as long as you're doing it for the benefit of the elder, nothing in care consultation is always true, just nearly always.

Don't Forget the Client's Family

There's a quote by Albert Einstein that's been going around for (too) many years: "The definition of insanity is doing the same thing over and over and expecting a different result." There are two things wrong with that quote. First, Einstein never said it. Second, doing the same thing over and over again and expecting a different result is not the definition of insanity, it's the definition of ineffectiveness.

Doubling down, by using a more authoritative voice (typically done, subconsciously), being repetitive, displaying impatience, and insisting that you and the expertise you rode in on knows better, will cause those who disagree with you to double down in turn.

The opposite of talking isn't listening. The opposite of talking is waiting.
—Fran Leibowitz

It's a given in social services that the key to being effective is to listen and understand. But though I should know better, I still fall in love with my voice and forget to listen to clients and their families. The urge to lecture, rather than listen and discuss, doesn't recede just because you (should) know better.

If you're experienced at any demanding endeavor—piano, Tai Chi, running, cooking, yoga—you know you can learn to take your skills for granted to the point that your good habits fall into less-good habits. When I practice Tai Chi in the morning, I do better when I remind myself to breathe, to go slow, or to remember to pay attention to a particular movement. In one of my meditation apps, the guide suggests that I use the occasional chime to refocus on my breathing. By using some object in the room to remind you to stay patient and listen, you can set a similar guide.

Now That I'm Listening, For What Do I Listen?

The first reason to listen carefully is simple: your clients and family feel heard. When there are diverse opinions among family members, or outright conflict, people fear that they won't be heard. It's likely that they've rehearsed their side of things and their point of view becomes important just because they're thinking about it. An approach I use is to take notes and summarize each point of view after everyone has had a chance to talk. It doesn't take that long, even if someone needs to clarify, and the result is that all participants feel heard and respected.

There are additional reasons I summarize after the contributions from participants. The participants may have been so focused on what they want to contribute, they forgot to listen to others. And they may change their opinions after considering the point of view of others. The change of opinion doesn't happen often, but it does happen.

Also keep in mind some people are more assertive than others, so you may have to elicit opinions from the reserved participants. Just because someone doesn't say something doesn't mean they don't have a point of view.

The second reason to listen carefully is to hear the language of the participant. The words people use can tell you how they feel about an issue, but more important, how they view the world. To change others, you must change yourself. That change will occur through understanding how others use language and changing your own to match theirs.

To give a simple example, if someone starts their statement with "I think," it's a losing proposition to change the language to "I feel."

(Therapists do this because they're big on feelings.) It's not your job to teach others your preferred ways of expressing points of view. Don't change them, change yourself.

Understanding how people express themselves and the cognitive frame behind that expression is an acquired skill. I can't emphasize too much to listen for the words people use to express their points of view. For instance, while they have the same meaning, I've carefully swapped *opinion* with *point of view.* The connotation of "opinion" is often *just* your opinion, but we understand and accept we have distinctive points of view. That simple difference in terms can change our—wait for it—point of view.

Chapter 19

Managing the Family Session

Preparation—Who's the Decision Maker?

If I avoid the above-described traffic jams of a family session, I have a clearer lane through the course of planning care. After affirming who's the client, I want to learn who's the decision-maker. Who will make the decisions regarding services for my client?

There are two types of decision-makers: (1) Legal. The elder's authority to make medical and financial decisions has been withdrawn. (2) In-effect. The elder may still be the legal decision maker, but he or she may have someone who strongly influences these decisions. It's the latter, the effective decision maker, who I'll be concerned with during the family sessions.

✻ Because he's capable, John, (my client) remains the legal decision maker regarding his financial and medical decisions. If John does become incapacitated, his son (as AIF) becomes the decision maker. But short of that, because he assists his father, financially, his son has influence over his father's decisions. For example, his son can interfere with John's medication. John's son is the effective decision maker.

✻ Linda, suffering from early Alzheimer's, is still the legal decision maker. Her daughter has arranged care, but that care has not addressed issues such as Linda's inability to prepare meals. However, they can't afford 24-hour care. The daughter manages finances and coordination of care and wants her mother to move into assisted living, but Linda refuses. Mother is the effective decision maker.

Deciding Where to Meet

When feasible, I prefer to hold family sessions in my office. It helps establish my role as an expert; it helps with focus; it does not favor the interests of any family member; I don't have to charge traveling time.

When elders are to be included, and their frailties make travel difficult, I will choose their home for the initial meeting. If only one family session is scheduled, that gives me the opportunity to assess elders in their living space.

When there are no turf issues or other conflicts among siblings, I'm comfortable meeting at the home of an adult child.

Creating Focus

Defining the issues is not just an opportunity to discuss the needs of my client, it's also a chance to learn how family members view the situation and how they deal with each other. Do they agree or disagree? The nature of conflict has many possibilities. Common contentions are one or more family members are doing more than their share, or one or more family members attempt to dominate the decisions, or there are disagreements regarding how much should be spent on services.

As we discuss and negotiate, I keep in mind, what are the essential decisions? For example, does the care giver need respite? Is the client still driving and driving unsafely? If so, what can be done? Are there home safety issues, such as a history of falls, a dangerous misuse of appliances, or wandering from the home? Are there legal issues, such as a client's reluctance to discuss attorney-in-fact?

Establish the Tone for the Session

Depending on how it's managed, the tone of a family session can be a trickle, a fountain, or a geyser of information and emotions. A trickle means members are being guarded, a geyser means family conflicts are being dumped into a pseudo-family therapy session. Like Goldilocks, I'm looking for just right, a steady fountain that doesn't flood the room.

During the initial family session, I note the familial relationships. Do the members feel they need to protect themselves, or do they trust each other? Is there a member that one or more members try to protect, or is there one who gets ganged up on? Does someone dominate or attempt to dominate the discussion and do others give in? Are members candid, or is there hidden agenda? Can participants joke, or is humor by you or a family member likely to be misunderstood?

Perhaps most important, who made the initial contact, why that person, and does he or she expect you (especially, if that person is paying you) to be their agent during family sessions? Once again, I communicate (indirectly, if possible) that I'm the agent of only the elder—a message that might need to be reinforced repeatedly. It may seem that I'm being unnecessarily repetitive (to both you and the family member who expects me to be their agent), but I am not. In my experience, this difference in perception is the primary source of conflicts.

* The daughter schedules a family session that includes her parents and her brother. Acting as the parents' care giver, her brother is living with their aging parents.

The daughter explains that there is a history of tension between her and her brother. He wishes to return to his own home and life, but she has been unsuccessful finding someone to take over the care giving. The sibling relationship is also strained because the brother is seen as the black sheep of the family and had struggles with alcohol abuse.

I use the above information as a guide to set the framework for the session. My first task is to ask the son about his care of his parents, elicit his concerns, and discuss his vision of a plan. This engages the son, validates his role as his parents' current care provider, and sets the tone for the session.

Establish Goals for the Session

While I make room for members to express their views and concerns regarding the elder, I avoid family drama by focusing on goals and being direct. This smooths the process and creates a model for everyone involved. I use phrases, such as "how do you see this affecting [an agreed upon goal]?"[1]

I start with at-risk issues, establish short- and long-term plans for care, and negotiate how each family member can participate in the elder's care. And I make sure that financial considerations are discussed.

Initial Phase

At the outset, I take control of the session, and when possible, plant the path to success even before the meeting takes place. I might issue a statement about that goal to each participant before the meeting and a statement early in the session—something like, "I'm glad we're all here to agree on, specifically, what each of us will do to make your mother's life better." I keep it simple to avoid a drift into conflict (or agreement) before everyone's been heard.

[1] Family therapists will recognize the choice of language to direct sessions.

I outline the issues the family should address. I listen to volunteered information as well as responses to my questions. And I note criticisms of my comments and suggestions, which are as useful as agreements.

I elicit involvement of all participants. I make sure everyone has the opportunity to discuss concerns.

I maintain the problem-solving focus. A family member may repeatedly complain of past hurts and attempt to get the group to address her anger towards her father. I acknowledge the hurt, then return the group to problem-solving.

I accept that the process may not please every family member. For example, the person who made the initial contact, such as the daughter, above, may be dissatisfied if I did not act as her agent.

I identify key issues. I ask the group if I've covered their concerns. However, I stay realistic about what can be accomplished in an initial session. I usually allow one and a half to two hours for each session but have a shorter session if the elder is present.

The conversation will be iterative. As the group discusses possible solutions, I review the progress, consider solutions to issues, and review the progress, again, until the family is satisfied for the time. The iteration will continue as long as I'm involved. Each attempt at a solution is an experiment to be evaluated, rather than a success or failure. I speak in language of trial, feedback, evaluation, new trial.

I provide education and coaching to the family and (if appropriate) to the elder to help them choose the best services. It's tempting to pretend to guide, while pushing hard for my preferences. But while candid about my preferences, I keep in mind that I'm the family's and client's consultant, not their boss. I accept with grace the choices families make when they differ from mine.[2] Families hire me for my expertise and usually want to follow my suggestions, but not always.

[2]I'm not always as graceful as I should be—it's another work-in-progress.

I keep the client at the forefront. My recommendations align with the wishes of the client, even when different from the goals of the family or of mine. Otherwise, I invite failure.

My recommendations are specific. For example, when recommending respite for the care giver, I specify the number of hours per day, per week, weekend overnights per month, a vacation each year, and so on.

I'm realistic. For example, I don't recommend respite away for a partner who prefers to stay at home.

My summary is specific. I make sure we agree, or that the decision makers are clear on what they'll do. We discuss who will follow up on each issue when multiple parties and issues are involved and decide if another family session is needed.

Agreements for Action

I never have all the facts, but I must make decisions and recommendations based on where we are in the process. Learning about your client is ongoing; I stay vigilant and keep an open mind.

Whether the family session has been contentious, congenial, or somewhere in between, I have two criteria for its success: (1) no one broke my furniture, and (2) we have come to a concrete agreement for who's going to do what. I do not end a family session without an agreement for concrete responsibilities.

The decisions and agreements should specify he'll do this, she'll do that, I'll do this and that. I state at the beginning that it can take several tries to get things going in the right direction.

After we've identified who will follow on each recommendation/ decision, I identify a contact person or persons for follow-up.

Chapter 20

How Family Sessions Go Bad

It's not a mystery when contentious family sessions don't result in progress. Look to these possibilities first:

- The participants do not arrive at *specific agreements* who would do what.
- You took sides, probably sub-consciously, in disagreements.
- You got caught up in the family drama. (See, above: you took sides.)
- One or more of the participants are not being honest. Often, it's because of family money and anticipated inheritance.

When there's conflict, it's hard to stay out of the family drama. I can't help (my human quality of) liking some family members more than others. Usually, my preferences come from who most takes to heart the best interests of my client. While understandable, my attitude is not helpful. My job is not to align with my favorites, but to get the optimum participation from all involved.

Part V

Working With Other Professionals

Chapter 21

Lawyers

Long-term Involvement

I work cooperatively with lawyers in a variety of ways, typically when we share a client over the long term, and the lawyer is also the client's attorney-in-fact (AIF).

* A woman in her mid-80s, without any surviving family, hires her lawyer as AIF. She has moved to an independent living facility with her now-deceased male companion. After being diagnosed with dementia, she moves to the facility's dementia care unit.

Her attorney hires a financial planner, a bill payer, and an accountant, and hires me for comprehensive care management.

My involvement is extensive: I schedule and attend all medical appointments and coordinate medical follow-up with dementia care staff; I put companion care services in place so my client can enjoy a variety of outings; and I find a counselor to work with my client on therapeutic life review.[1]

As the client's lawyer is the decision-maker, the two of us review my recommendations that are designed to enhance our client's quality of

[1] Reviewing with clients, their lifetime memories, using photos and other memorabilia to enhance understanding and comfort.

life. I follow this client until her passing, even planning and attending her memorial service.

* A woman in her 80s, born in Australia, married a U.S. citizen and moved with him to the U.S. Both had adult children from previous marriages, who still lived in their homelands. Her husband was her AIF, and when he passed, their lawyer assumed that role.

Diagnosed with dementia, she's living in an assisted living facility, when her lawyer/AIF hires me. I provide care management and create a plan for her to return to Australia, where she would be looked after by her adult daughter.

Multiple Lawyers' Involvement

Because they specialize or wish to avoid a conflict of interest, more than one lawyer may be involved in a care manager's work with a particular client.

* Following the death of her husband, an 88-year-old woman (Alice), who resides in an assisted living facility, hires a lawyer to update her will.

Because Alice has advancing dementia, her attorney is concerned that she does not have a trustworthy candidate to assign an AIF. Neither Alice nor her attorney trust her only living relative (her nephew) as an AIF candidate. Alice is concerned that both her nephew and her current living facility might exploit her considerable wealth. Along with the need for a will and AIF, Alice wishes to move to a different facility.

Alice hires me to assist with finding a facility that can better meet her needs and to help her find a suitable AIF to serve as her medical and financial decision maker. Alice's lawyer and I find an elder-law attorney who agrees to become her AIF, and I work with Alice to contract with the lawyer. In addition, I work with Alice's primary physician to get a document stating that, although diagnosed with dementia, she still has the capacity to make decisions about her medical care and choice of AIF.

After Alice agrees to assign AIF to the second lawyer, I schedule and accompany Alice to an appointment with a third lawyer (to avoid a conflict of interest) who, with the document from Alice's physician, and following a lengthy private conversation with Alice, completes the DPOA document that assigns the AIF.

Throughout the remainder of her life, Alice's lawyer/AIF and I work together to ensure that Alice has the best possible care in the most appropriate settings.

Brief Involvement

Often, a care consultant's collaboration with a lawyer is limited.

* My client is updating her planning documents that include her living will. Her lawyer asks that I assist in drafting the living will, as it's important that the instructions include those that she has already outlined in the Physician's Order for Life Sustaining Treatment (POLST). The POLST, completed by patients with the assistance of their primary physician, in addition to stating their choice to be resuscitated or not if heart and/or breathing cease, addresses specific medical interventions, such as hydration, tube feeding and antibiotic use. In contrast to the POLST, the living will typically addresses only this: if there is no chance of recovery from an illness, does an individual want to be sustained on life support?

Because my client had a relative who, with tube feeding, lived for more than a year and maintained a satisfactory quality of life, my client decides, if tube feeding becomes necessary, she will try it. Based on my client's Physician's Order for Life Sustaining Treatment (POLST), I provide a draft for my client's lawyer to use in the living will.

✻ A lawyer's client (Bill) has been coordinating medical care and providing home care to his mother, now deceased.

The lawyer is assisting Bill in the determination of the mother's estate and division of assets between Bill and his brother, the other heir to the estate. Bill's care allowed their mother to remain in her home until the end of her life—that is, she did not have to spend funds for professional home care—and Bill wants to be compensated from the estate.

The lawyer hires me to write a report that summarizes the cost for services if they had been provided by a licensed homecare agency. My report is used to assist in obtaining compensation for his client.

✻ The only son (who is AIF) hires me for his father, who is suffering from advanced dementia, multiple health issues, and need for assistance with daily personal care. I coordinate home care, medical care, and work with them throughout my client's hospitalization and death.

The son, emotionally and financially dependent on his father, is devastated by his father's passing. He is on disability and has been living with his father.

He is ill-equipped to address the resolution of his father's estate. After his father dies, he hires me to assist in finding and hiring a lawyer to address resolution of the estate. At the son's request, I coordinate and attend his appointment with a lawyer, take notes for the son's reference, and ensure that he has his questions answered.

✻ The daughter (and AIF) of an elderly woman with advanced dementia has moved her mother to an adult family home. It was her mother's wish to remain in her home, but the daughter places her in an adult family home because she could not find affordable home care that her mother required. Because her mother would wander from her house, day or night, she needs expensive 24-hour supervision.

The AIF's brother, *successor* (back-up) as AIF, is unhappy with his sister's decision and has hired an attorney to challenge it. The AIF hires me to assess their mother's care needs, to assess the adult family home, and research potential cost of available round-the-clock care options if her mother is returned to her home. She also asks that I speak with her brother's lawyer and meet with her brother to understand his concerns.

On the phone, the brother's lawyer conveys his client's concerns, and adds that his client might initiate guardianship proceedings if the siblings aren't able to resolve their disagreement.

I provide a written assessment and recommendations to the siblings and their attorneys, followed by a meeting with the siblings. Following the meeting, the siblings agree to keep their mother in the adult family home.

Chapter 22

Doctors

At the request of the client, the client's AIF, or on occasion, a family member, I often attend my client's medical appointments. Because physicians' schedules limit their time with patients, I make the most of these appointments by preparing questions and documenting answers that can be referenced by the client, family members, and me. I also make sure that nothing important gets lost between my client's physician and (when applicable) the medical staff at assisted living facilities. While the doctor's office sends a summary of the visit, I augment the report with a discussion with the facility medical staff.

While much of my involvement with physicians deals with common maladies and concerns, the following examples focus on the less common. My involvement ranges from the simple to the complex.

* I'm hired by a client's attorney-in-fact (AIF) to accompany a client to her consultation with a surgeon, regarding possible neck surgery. Jill's AIF is concerned that the surgery is unwarranted.

I assist Jill to question the surgeon, especially, whether surgery is necessary. Following the appointments, I email summaries to Jill and her AIF. Jill and her AIF will decide whether to proceed with the surgery.

I accompany Jill to several appointments with the surgeon and an appointment for a second opinion. Again, I email summaries of each appointment to Jill and her AIF. Following, I answer any additional questions.

Jill and her AIF decide to proceed with the surgery. I'm present for the duration of the six-hour procedure and provide email updates to the AIF, who is unavailable to be present. I attend all follow-up appointments.

* My client, Dot, who suffers from dementia, lives alone in her multi-level home. Her hygiene is poor because she forgets to bathe, and she has lost the ability to plan, purchase, and prepare meals. Her refrigerator is full of expired foods and spoiled leftovers, leaving her with a diet primarily of ice cream and sweets. When she takes the stairs to her laundry room, she is at risk for a fall.

Dot does not understand the risks of living alone and wishes to continue living on her own. Her AIF (her nephew) lives four hours away, so is unable to provide sufficient supervision. A neighbor helps Dot, but her AIF is concerned that the neighbor might exploit Dot financially.

Because of our concerns, her AIF and I enlist Dot's physician to help with a transition to a dementia care facility. Her physician agrees that Dot no longer has the capacity to make decisions and that 24-hour assistance is necessary. She completes the admission paperwork and helps us explain to Dot the scheduled move.

* Ninety-five-year-old Anna, aided by her physician, has completed her document, the Physician's Order for Life Sustaining Treatment (POLST). Her daughter, Maggie, who is her AIF, persuades Anna to convey her desire for full resuscitation if her heart and breathing cease. Though diagnosed with dementia, Anna is capable to make this decision.

Later, when Anna is referred to hospice care, Maggie persuades her mother to refuse, because the hospice agency requires a status of "do *not* resuscitate" in her POLST. Following a 911 call, Anna is hospitalized, and the hospital physician believes that death is imminent. Anna is no longer capable to make decisions, and as AIF, Maggie insists that tube feeding be started.

In a meeting with the hospital social worker and me, Maggie refuses to change Anna's POLST status. Following, the hospital physician contacts me to discuss a referral to the hospital ethics board. He wants to spare Anna the pain and spare the hospital staff the trauma of attempting to resuscitate a dying patient.

Previously, I had arranged a meeting with Anna, Maggie, and their minister to discuss end-of-life care. I contact this minister, who follows with a phone call to the hospital physician and then to Maggie. The minister persuades Maggie to change Anna's code status and Anna dies peacefully within two days.

* Susan is suffering from dementia and multiple medical issues. Her impairments result in hospitalizations and discharges to either skilled rehabilitation facilities or to her home accompanied by home care.

Most care facilities require an activated power of attorney to allow the AIF to make medication, surgery, and discharge-planning decisions, when the resident is no longer capable to make these decisions. After accompanying Susan to several medical appointments, I believe it is time for the durable power of attorney (DPOA) to be activated, which results in the appointment of the attorney-in-fact.

DPOA's are often written so they can be activated by only a written statement from the physician: "The patient is no longer capable to make medical, care, and financial decisions."

Years earlier, Susan had assigned AIF to a trusted family member, who hired me to manage Susan's care. I advise the AIF to write a letter to the physician requesting the necessary statement. At the scheduled appointment, the physician, Susan, and I discuss the transfer of decision-making authority. The physician then writes the letter to activate the power of attorney.

* Alan, who suffers from dementia, has yet to complete DPOA documents. His lawyer thought it was time, but unlike Susan (above),

Alan does not have a trusted family member or friend to fill the role of AIF.

I ask his physician to assess whether Alan is capable to assign an AIF. The physician has worked with Alan for many years and believes, despite Alan's advancing dementia, he's able to make informed decisions about his medical care. The physician's statement to that effect means Alan can assign AIF to a lawyer of his choice.

* The daughter of my client (Anthony) initiates a claim for home care benefits through Anthony's long-term care policy. His home care consists of a care giver providing assistance a few days a week. The care giver helps with shopping, meal preparation, and medication reminders. With this minimal assistance, Anthony is independent.

Anthony, a smoker, is diagnosed with chronic obstructive pulmonary disease (COPD) and needs 24-hour assistance from an oxygen tank. He continues to smoke and often forgets to resume the oxygen after smoking. The smoking creates a health and safety issue, and to address it, his daughter wishes to increase care.

After Anthony's physician submits the paperwork to support the need for increased home care, the long-term health insurance company sends a nurse to assess Anthony's situation. Anthony performs too well on a mini mental status exam (MMSE) to qualify for additional home care.

I consult with Anthony's physician, who explains that Anthony's cognitive status depends on the level of oxygen in his blood. Following, his physician administers another MMSE, which demonstrates cognitive impairment. The physician re-submits this documentation, his assessment, and recommendations. The claim is approved.

I haven't always gotten the outcomes I desired when working with physicians. The following example illustrates the importance of persistence.

* Ninety-one-year-old Natalie is living in an apartment in an assisted living facility. Though suffering from dementia, she uses routine and a structured environment to maintain her independence.

Subsequently, she suffers a fall and breaks her hip, which requires a hip replacement. From the hospital, Natalie is transferred to a skilled nursing facility for rehabilitation.

The injuries from the fall add physical impairment to Natalie's cognitive impairment, and her care in her previous setting becomes inadequate. Her daughter, who as attorney-in-fact makes all Natalie's medical and financial decisions, agrees that Natalie should move to an adult family home.

Natalie's transition to the adult family home is rocky. She is used to the independence and privacy in her own residence and experiences her new living situation as intrusive. She is also confused about where she's living and why she now needs so much attention from care givers. Because Natalie is kind and gracious, she responds with agitation, rather than resistance. She becomes so agitated that she stays awake all night. Sleeplessness exacerbates her agitation and interferes with recovery from the surgery.

I accompany Natalie to an appointment with her primary physician, with the hope that she will prescribe anti-anxiety medication and/or an anti-depressant to assist Natalie to sleep. To my dismay, her physician states that anti-depressants and anti-anxiety meds are not her choice for those suffering from dementia and prescribes anti-psychotic meds instead.

I have experienced the opposite response for those suffering from dementia: poor outcomes with anti-psychotic meds and positive outcomes when anti-anxiety and anti-depressant meds are used to alleviate sleeplessness. I have seen this with several clients and even with my own mother.

There are situations where more potent sedating meds (an anti-psychotic) are necessary, such as when clients physically abuse care givers, but this is not the case with Natalie. I tactfully question the physician, and in retrospect, I wish I had been more assertive. She prescribes an anti-psychotic medicine that sets in motion a miserable but avoidable sequence.

Although Natalie's sleep improves, her daytime agitation increases, and Natalie begins to strike care givers. Alarmed, I attempt to get the meds changed, but as a nurse acts as intermediary, my communication with the physician is impeded. The doctor does not make a change, so I ask the nurse for an in-home mental health consultation.

A nurse practitioner comes to the adult family home to evaluate Natalie. She explains that in her experience some elderly patients become more agitated on anti-psychotic meds,[1] and this is what she thinks is happening. However, the nurse's role does not include making medication recommendations. She can only relate what she observes. Her verbal report through the nurse and written report to the physician fall on deaf ears.

Natalie's agitation increases to where she is trying to get up from her chair without assistance, which puts her at increased risk for another fall. I immediately contact her physician. Again, I have to go through the nurse rather than talk to the doctor. This is on a Friday, and when the day ends without a response, I'm directed by her nurse to contact the on-call doctor. I'm stunned when the on-call doctor, following my description of the history of my client's symptoms, recommends increasing the anti-psychotic medication. I respond by informing the doctor that Natalie's daughter (the AIF) will not agree to the increase. The on-call doctor refuses to make any other change in Natalie's medications.

Natalie's daughter and I have already discussed the option of her refusing the anti-psychotic medication on her mother's behalf. Given that there will be nothing to replace the anti-psychotic medication to address her mother's agitation, this is a difficult decision. Before any decisions or changes can be made, Natalie has another fall, breaks her other hip and is hospitalized for emergency surgery. In the hospital,

[1] In other words, she agrees with me

because it has likely contributed to her fall, we are able to finally get her off the anti-psychotic medication.

* While, on occasion, I've had differences with physicians, I've also worked with terrific doctors. I've been accompanying Lillian to appointments with her primary physician for almost three years. As he had been the physician for her husband, before the husband's death, Lillian has known her doctor for many years and has a warm and playful relationship with him. It is a pleasure to be a part of the joking and singing that they enjoy together.

Lillian's primary medical issues are dementia, high blood pressure, and atrial fibrillation. She has a pacemaker to regulate her heart rhythm. On a routine follow-up visit, the doctor observes unusually low blood pressure and an irregular heart beat. An electrocardiogram confirms his readings.

Immediately, he contacts Lillian's cardiologist and coordinates admission to Lillian's preferred hospital. The hospital is just across the street, so rather than call 911, her doctor drives Lillian and me to the emergency entrance. While he waits with Lillian in his car, I enter the hospital to alert staff, who are ready with a wheelchair to admit Lillian.

Chapter 23

Social Workers

Introduction

As a care consultant, I frequently interact with other social workers. Their interests for your clients, stated or not, may differ from yours. Yours stem from your deep knowledge of your clients and the best possible quality of life for their future. Social workers employed by institutions must divide their concerns between helping your client and looking out for the interests of their employer, whether the bottom line or otherwise.

Social workers practice in a variety of institutional settings. For example, they coordinate discharges from hospitals and skilled nursing facilities, usually sending patients back to their home or to a higher level of care. In their roles in senior centers, day health programs, and home health and hospice, social workers provide information about and coordinate access to community programs and resources.

The above tasks of institutional social workers are similar to those of a care consultant. We both facilitate transitions and access to services. The differences lie in the level of advocacy, time and effort, and familiarity with each client's situation. Because I have ongoing oversight, I can correct mistaken assumptions. Sometimes, the overlap of responsibilities and different interests leads to a clash. I've been accused of trespassing, more than once: "That's my job! Your services are unnecessary. I provide the same services for free." But because of my superior knowledge of my clients, I persevere to guide the discharge planning.

While, within their institutional constraints, most social workers will show concern for your client, don't expect the same from the bill-payer, that is, the health insurance company. Their goal is to move your client from the more expensive institution to the cheaper one. The shorter the potential stay at the current setting, the more quickly I get involved with the transition.

To work with the social worker, I get a release of information signed by my client or my client's decision maker. When I work with an attorney-in-fact or guardian, I request permission to consult with the social worker on the client's behalf.

I prepare for case conferences with a list of issues that my client is experiencing and ask how these issues will be addressed.

In a skilled rehabilitation setting, case conferences will include nurses, and physical, occupational, and speech therapists. They will report on your client's progress and whether your client is expected to achieve their previous level of functioning.

Hospital case conferences are rare and involve fewer staff. The case conference will include a projected discharge date and services and equipment to be ordered on discharge. Given the relatively short stay, I connect with the social worker early to plan the transition.

Social Workers' Practice Settings

Note: All references to Medicare eligibility are based on regulations that were current at the time the following examples occurred. Regulations change. See https://www.medicare.gov for current Medicare coverage and regulations.

Hospitals

Discharge planners are under pressure to get their patients out of the hospital before their insurance runs out. Medicare pays for a maximum number of days for each diagnosis treated,[1] and the hospital must stay within these limits unless complications arise.

Skilled nursing facilities

Social workers in skilled nursing facilities (SNFs) that accept medicare are under similar though less urgent pressure to plan patient discharge. Medicare can cover patients in a SNF if they meet the criteria of receiving skilled care and are making progress toward goals.

The SNF is responsible to arrange a "safe" discharge, and it's the social worker's job to make that happen. The patient should be discharged to a setting where they'll obtain needed care. This may be back to their home with in-home services and adaptive equipment or a transfer to a setting that will provide additional care. If necessary, the patient will continue at the SNF; when their medicare eligibility runs out, the patient becomes responsible for payment.

Adult day health

Social workers in an adult day health setting often guide initial visits for potential clients. They may present alternatives if adult day health is inappropriate.

Senior center

Senior center social workers' responsibilities align with the services their center offers. If the center offers programs that support seniors' health and well-being, such as the Program to Encourage Active Rewarding Lives for Seniors (PEARLS), the social worker will screen candidates and

[1]Again, check https://www.medicare.gov for current Medicare coverage and regulations.

may take part in the PEARLS sessions. The social worker also provides resource information to the center's members.

In home, Medicare funded

Medicare covers in-home skilled health services, if the Medicare recipient is considered "homebound."[2]

Skilled home health services, such as nursing or physical therapy, may be ordered following a rehabilitation stay. As these health providers work with the client, they may identify a need for additional services and ask the primary physician to order a social worker to visit the client's home to discuss services in the community.

Hospice

Hospice social workers provide resource information to patients and their families. Often they discuss all services offered by hospice and help to coordinate these services. They also provide information on services available from other sources.

Coordinating with institutional social workers

✻ My client, suffering from dementia and congestive heart failure, is undergoing an examination by his physician. After noting the client's severe edema and a pulse of 150, she sends him to the emergency room, and he's subsequently hospitalized. Following treatment, discharge is being planned. I schedule to meet with my client, his wife, daughter, and other family members at the hospital to discuss and coordinate the discharge.

When I arrive at the hospital, I have the social worker paged and request a meeting to discuss recommendations and options with my

---

[2]Homebound criteria listed in the 2019, *Medicare Handbook*: *(1) You have trouble leaving your home without help (like using a cane, wheelchair or walker, or crutches; special transportation; or help from another person) because of an injury or illness. (2) Leaving your home isn't recommended because of your condition. (3) You're normally unable to leave your home because it's a major effort.*

client and his family. The social worker advises that my client is eligible for a skilled nursing facility (SNF) and prints out a list from medicare.gov of Medicare-certified nursing homes in the area that have openings. I narrow the family's choices by explaining the nursing home certification process (i.e., Medicare's rating system) and the rehabilitation services he will receive during his stay.

* David is admitted to the hospital with an elevated temperature, dehydration, and atrial fibrillation. With treatment with IV fluids and antibiotics, his temperature is stabilized. Because of David's advanced dementia, he no longer has the capacity to make decisions about his care. On David's admission, the hospital contacts his son, the attorney-in-fact. His son, who lives out of state, has hired me as his father's care manager and gives the hospital permission to work with me.

After three days in the hospital, David is eligible for discharge to a skilled nursing facility (SNF) to start rehabilitation. I provide the social worker with a list of acceptable SNFs (based on Medicare certification ratings), their proximity to David's local family, and my previous experience with the facilities. The social worker contacts these SNFs to check for openings, consults with me on the final decision, and arranges the transfer of paperwork and the patient.

* Andy is hospitalized following a fall. Staff at his assisted living facility find him lying next to his bed and believe consumption of alcohol contributed to the fall.

I visit Andy in the hospital, and he is unclear where he is and where he has been living. Andy has not been diagnosed with dementia and has not previously exhibited this level of cognitive impairment. I discuss this with the hospital social worker and request he inform the hospital physician. The physician orders testing for cognitive impairment.

Advocacy with institutional social workers

* Grace is hospitalized with low blood pressure and atrial fibrillation.

She suffers from dementia and receives assistance with medications and is cared for in a retirement community.

Before her hospitalization, the facility staff noted that Grace has discontinued her personal training sessions and spends an increasing amount of time in bed. Her appetite has declined and she has to be accompanied to the dining room.

Grace's attorney-in-fact gives me permission to work with the hospital social worker on the discharge plan. Her cardiologist oversees her three-day stay at the hospital.

The hospital social worker believes that Grace's cognitive impairment means Grace can't follow instructions sufficiently to benefit from skilled rehabilitation. The hospital physical therapist recommends a discharge to home with in-home physical therapy.

Because of her decline before hospitalization, I advocate for a transfer to a SNF for rehabilitation. My arguments to the social worker are as follows: My client has been able to follow the instructions of a personal trainer. She has suffered a decline and is now at risk for future falls. In-home physical therapy would provide only two sessions per week rather than daily therapy in a SNF, and daily therapy could help Grace return to her previous physical condition.

Before Grace is allowed to return to her retirement community, the wellness director needs to make an assessment of Grace's condition. Unfortunately, the wellness director is new to the facility and to my client. She approves Grace's return, with the limited twice-weekly in-home physical therapy.

The physical therapy proves insufficient, and Grace continues to decline. She spends most of her time in bed and struggles to walk to meals, even with staff assistance. The wellness director eventually agrees that a rehabilitation stay is in Grace's best interest. Grace's doctor orders skilled rehabilitation, and I arrange the admission. Since Grace has been out of the hospital for less than a month, she is still eligible for Medicare to cover the rehabilitation facility.

* Barton is a developmentally disabled 62-year-old man, who lives independently in his home. I have been hired by a family member because of concerns about Barton's poor nutrition, weight loss, decreased activity, observed strength, and social isolation. Barton has a history of depression but did not like the anti-depressants prescribed, and they have been discontinued at his request.

Barton spends most days watching TV. He is capable of taking bus rides to his doctor, for shopping, and to visit family. I help Barton join the nearby senior center. At my suggestion, Barton tries an exercise class but is not motivated to regularly attend.

The senior center offers a depression management program (PEARLS) for free to their members. I schedule a screening appointment with the social worker in charge of the program and attend the appointment with Barton. Because of his answers related to his mood, Barton does not qualify for the program.

I ask for a second meeting with the social worker. She agrees to check in with Barton regularly to offer support and encouragement.

* Alice is discharged from the hospital with orders for home health nursing and physical therapy. During the intake for the home services, the nurse asks Alice (who is currently living in an assisted living community) if she would like a social worker to present additional assisted living options. For reasons I'll explain below, Alice is interested.

Alice is a 58-year-old woman with multiple diagnoses, including insulin-dependent diabetes and congestive heart failure. I have been her care manager for over five years and have worked with the wellness director of Alice's living facility to set up nurse oversight of her diabetes. Before the oversight was set up, Alice had done a poor job of managing her insulin and experienced multiple life-threatening incidents.

While Alice appreciates the independence and privacy of her apartment in the assisted living community, she still wants to manage the insulin on her own. As I know Alice has requested the meeting in hope she'd find a facility that will allow her to self-manage her insulin, I want to be present at her meeting with the social worker.

I'm taken aback when the social worker proposes an adult family home as ideal. The social worker presents life in an adult family home as akin to when Alice shared a house with fellow students on her college campus. I counter the social worker's idealized version with a realistic one, and explain the care and medication management the staff would provide. I make it clear to Alice that she would have a lot less privacy and independence than she enjoys in her current apartment. Alice declines further visits from the social worker.

Chapter 24

Out of Area and Out of State Care Consultants

On occasion, I'm hired to arrange a move of a client into my practice area or a move of a client out of my practice area. When moving a client to my area, a face to face assessment is not possible, so I rely on information from family and from professionals in the client's current location. It's helpful when my client or client's attorney-in-fact agrees to hire a care consultant at their end who I can confer with regarding the move. Likewise, when a care consultant is hired in the area where my client is moving to, I have confidence the change will go smoothly.

✻ Thomas, the only child and the attorney-in-fact of Gwen, a 76 year-old widowed woman who lives out of state, seeks my assistance for his mother. Gwen is recovering from a stroke and is undergoing rehabilitation in a skilled nursing facility (SNF). Before her stroke, Gwen had been living in her own home.

Gwen's lack of motivation for physical therapy slows her recovery. Her appetite is poor, which leads to weight loss. She refuses to participate in activities and spends most of her time in bed. Gwen's physician prescribes an anti-depressant.

A year before the stroke, Gwen invited a woman and her boyfriend to live in her home to help with chores, run errands, and provide transportation. Thomas visited Gwen several times during that year and has reason to believe his mother is being taken advantage of financially by this couple. Following the stroke, this couple continues to live in Gwen's home and visit Gwen at the SNF. Gwen tells her son that the couple wants her to return home as soon as possible. Thomas suspects the couple is concerned with their own interests at the expense of his mother's.

Thomas hires me to help arrange his mother's move from her home in Oregon to an adult family home in his home state, which is also the state of my practice. Contact with the social worker at the SNF confirms that Gwen will require a significant amount of home care or a move to a facility that provides 24/7 care. Given the complicating factors of Gwen's recent stroke, her depression, and the questionable involvement of the couple, I recommend that Thomas hire a care consultant who practices near Gwen to complete an assessment, provide support to Gwen at the SNF, and help coordinate the planned move from that end.

I locate and interview a care consultant near Gwen's current residence, and Thomas hires her. The care consultant's assessment confirms that Gwen's low motivation hinders her recuperation. While details of the move are being finalized, I recommend that Thomas hire a companion to visit his mother in the SNF, three times a week, to assist her with the activities in the facility. The companion's visits help Gwen recuperate sufficiently to make the move.

Subsequently, Gwen moves to an adult family home near her son. With the support from her son, the structure and care provided by the adult family home, and the physical and occupational therapies, Gwen's mood improves, and her appetite and strength return.

* Alex's father, Raymond, is an 86 year-old man suffering from dementia. Raymond lives in a retirement community that offers elegant evening meals in a communal dining room but no assistance with

personal care or medication management. Residents who need these services have to hire private care givers.

Alex lives a two-hour drive from his father's retirement community so is unable to assist Raymond in managing his essential needs, such as daily medication and medical appointments. Alex hires me to coordinate the needed care. When it becomes clear that the amount of daily oversight Raymond requires is too expensive, Alex decides to move Raymond to an assisted living facility near Alex's home, which will take Raymond out of my practice area.

I assist the transition to the new facility and recommend that a care consultant be hired to oversee care for Raymond in the new setting. I interview three prospects, summarize their costs, qualifications, and approaches. I convey the information to Alex who makes his selection.

✻ Agnes lives alone in her own home. She suffers from dementia and is at risk due to difficulties with medication management, self care, nutrition, and driving. Agnes' daughter, Tracy, lives across the country and hires me to complete an assessment and make recommendations for her mother's care. Based on my assessment, Tracy decides to move her mother to Tracy's home town. Tracy has been considering such a move and has contacted a local care consultant for information about assisted living settings. My assessment and recommendations are shared with the local care consultant, and Tracy requests that the care consultant and I discuss the options for care for Agnes. Following, the care consultant assists Tracy with the selection of a care setting.

✻ I'm contacted by Allison, the daughter of a couple who wishes to move closer to Allison. Allison's mother, Celia, hired a local care consultant before the couple's decision to move, and subsequently hires me to coordinate care in their new setting.

Celia's husband suffers from dementia and has been moved to the dementia care unit of their current retirement community. Celia asks me to confer with their local care consultant to assist with their move to a retirement community, near Allison, that offers assisted living and dementia care.

After her husband passes away, Celia decides she wants to return to her home state, where several of her friends and her son lives. Her son helps locate an assisted care setting, and I recommend that Celia re-hire her previous care consultant. Celia has experienced physical decline, and following discussions with me, the care consultant coordinates the necessary level of care that will be provided in the new setting.

Chapter 25

Financial Services

I occasionally work with those who provide financial services to my clients.

Trustees, as the name implies, oversee expenditures from a trust. The trust may have been established for a disabled adult of now deceased parents. Typically, the trustee is identified in the trust and is a relative or a professional trust company.

Financial advisers focus on investments for clients.

Bill payers are hired by clients or their attorney-in-fact when clients are either no longer capable of handling their own bills or just want help with bill paying.

* I'm contacted by the financial adviser for a couple. Both members of the couple are undergoing cognitive and physical decline, and according to the financial adviser, are making poor financial decisions. They have suddenly sold their home and are renting, while searching for a home in which to live out their lives. They are ignoring the recommendations for the care assistance they each need, while paying a large salary to a young woman to run errands.

Concerned about their poor money management, and worried that they might choose a home that will not take into account their infirmities, the financial adviser persuades them to hire a care manager to do an assessment and make recommendations on their current and future care.

I outline the current home care they need and project their needs as they continue to decline. I encourage them to buy a home close to medical services and one that can be adapted for safety and future home care.

✻ My client is residing in an assisted living facility and has help with medication management and bathing. Despite the support of his daughter, he's no longer able to manage his finances and can't account for large purchases. I advise that he hire a bill payer to pay his bills and prepare statements for tax purposes.

✻ A middle-aged disabled woman, supported by a trust fund, is referred to me because of multiple medical and care issues. My client's finances are overseen by a financial planner, a bill payer, and the trustee who is also the attorney-in-fact and my client's sister. My client and her trustee make all decisions related to major medical and care expenses. My role is to obtain the information from involved physicians to inform these decisions.

Chapter 26

Guardians

Thanksgiving, Christmas, and Super Bowls come just once a year. Thankfully, in my practice, guardianships come even less often.[1] As my lawyer friend and sometimes colleague tells it, taking away someone's adult rights is demeaning and should be the last resort in dealing with an adult suffering from cognitive impairment.

My involvements with guardianships stem primarily from disagreements between clients' adult children—usually a dispute over what's best for their parent. The result of the proceedings is typically that one of the siblings is assigned guardianship.

I get hired when the arguments continue after the court proceedings are finished.

* Because of her advanced dementia, Gladys has been deemed incapacitated by the judge. Her adult children, Cal and Audrey, both seek guardianship, and the court sides with Audrey. The court determines that Cal had exerted undue influence over his mother's decisions about her care and about expenses to ensure her care.

The judge orders Cal's visits to be supervised, and Audrey's attorney recommends that a care consultant be hired to supervise the visits. I

[1]A guardian is a court-appointed protector of an incapacitated person.

meet with Audrey to obtain background information, meet with Gladys at her dementia care facility, and meet with Cal right before the first supervised visit.

* Philip files and wins guardianship for their mother, Lois, largely because of his sister's (Violet) interference with Lois' care.

Lois lives in an assisted care facility. The facility has sought a restraining order against Violet, due to her abusive treatment of their care staff, and because of Lois' agitation during and following Violet's visits.

Lois loves her daughter and wants to continue their visits. Because of Violet's strange behavior and her poor relationship with her brother, it's inadvisable for Philip to supervise these visits, so Philip hires me to supervise them at a neutral location.

After Philip and I agree on a location, he coordinates the logistics of the participation among the three of us.

* Thomas is his father's attorney-in-fact, and because of his father's advancing dementia, his guardian. While Thomas' brother, Lee, did not contest the guardianship, he becomes unhappy with the cost of their father's home care. Thomas believes that Lee's concern for the cost is because Lee is struggling financially and wants some help with his bills.

Thomas requests a comprehensive written assessment of the care required to maintain their father in their father's own home.

Thomas takes seriously his responsibility that their father have the best quality of life that his significant assets allow him. He hires me to confirm that the care provided is not only necessary but also enhances their father's life as much as possible.

Chapter 27

Counselors

The professional education of many care consultants is in counseling or counseling-focused social work. A counseling background can provide experience to assist clients to negotiate difficult and stressful decision making about their futures, especially when families are involved. Counseling skills help you lead family sessions about a client's care and how family members might support the aging process.

The downside of a counseling background is that it can hijack your focus as a care consultant. To aid my own focus as well as the family's, I make our task clear at the outset of the meeting. (See Part IV, Working with Families.)

Your knowledge and training in counseling will also tell you when a referral to a counselor is appropriate.

* A middle-aged single adult, with multiple health issues and living in an assisted living facility, suffers from anxiety and depression related to her steady physical decline. Anti-depressant medications have not helped, and (talk) therapy has been tried in the past but discontinued by the client. I recommend that she return to counseling and assist her to find a counselor who accepts her insurance.

* A single adult, with a history of alcohol abuse, tries Alcoholics Anonymous but does not feel comfortable with their format. I research

and find a nearby counselor who specializes in drug and alcohol abuse counseling and will accept my client's insurance.

* A couple moves in with their two adult daughters. To ease the burden on the daughters, the couple seeks consultation with me on their own. One member of the couple suffers from mild cognitive impairment and related depression. I recommend individual counseling to help with adjustment to the cognitive impairment and with the new living arrangements.

* A couple who run a family business grapples with the wife's recent physical and cognitive decline. The wife's decline has shifted all household and business responsibilities to her husband, which puts stress on him and on their relationship. I refer them to a marriage counselor.

Chapter 28

Assisted Living and Dementia Care

While modern medicine may extend a person's life, it doesn't necessarily extend the ability to manage one's own care. As a result, we have seen a rapid growth of assisted living and dementia care facilities.

Care Facilities

Retirement and assisted living

Retirement living in a for-profit facility typically includes these services: rental of an apartment, one to two meals a day, snacks, transportation for errands and medical appointments, housekeeping and room maintenance, changing and washing of linens, and an activity program. To the above, *assisted living* adds any or all additional services: a third meal, laundry service, medication management, bathing and dressing assistance, escort to meals, wellness checks, scheduled toileting assistance, and incontinence care. Such facilities expect their residents to be capable of moving from standing to sitting, and vice versa (known as *transfers*). Assisted living facilities may provide scheduled (but not on-call) help to move within the resident's apartment.

If a resident requires additional services, an assisted living nurse meets with the resident and develops a *negotiated care plan* that describes the provided services, the schedule, and their cost. Facilities typically review the care plan after a month and then every six months or annually. The care plan is also updated as needed, such as following a hospitalization.

Dementia care

As those who suffer from dementia are at risk for social isolation, some facilities have day programs that provide structure, stimulation, and social interaction. These programs can also provide respite for a higher-functioning member of a couple who's providing care for a spouse.

Those with dementia may also need additional safety measures. Some large retirement/assisted living facilities offer *secure* dementia care. The unit is locked, with a code or keys for staff to enter and exit. Secure dementia care is most appropriate for those who need 24-hour supervision.

Continuing care retirement communities

Unlike retirement and assisted living, continuing care retirement communities (CCRC) provide a continuum of services that include independent living, assisted living, and within this single community, skilled nursing care. Models vary whether retirement and assisted living are integrated or are provided in separate areas of the community. Skilled nursing care is separated from the private apartments.

Staffing

Retirement/assisted living communities and CCRCs have large staffs. I identify and work with the appropriate staff to coordinate my client's care and activities. I monitor staff turnover and how it may affect my client's care. With the large staff and large turnover, if I'm not vigilant, the procedures and coordination we've agreed on can fall by the wayside. (I go into more detail, below.)

Assisted living services are managed by the wellness director, a nurse who oversees services to all residents who require assistance with medication management and personal care.

The wellness director meets with the resident to set up or review the negotiated care plan. I usually attend the initial and subsequent meetings to review the agreement, advocate for needed changes, and clarify the cost.

The activities director (often called *vitality director*) oversees two resident services. Their responsibility includes the practical needs of transportation to medical appointments, shopping, other outings, and additional activities, such as exercise programs and arts and crafts. And they oversee the exercise classes geared toward the particular population, which may take place in a swimming pool (if available) and in an on-site gym.

The coordination of transportation to appointments is especially important for clients who are unable to keep track of their own schedules. The activities director also encourages residents to participate in activities that they enjoy.

Maintenance services make sure all building systems, such as heating, and cable and internet connections, are working. The maintenance supervisor can be especially helpful when a client is moving into the facility or moving to another apartment within the facility.

Concierge services are sometimes offered by assisted living facilities. These services can include arrangement of private transportation, co-ordination of deliveries to the resident, and personal assistance with access to amenities in the facility.

✣ My client has a full schedule of medical appointments and is unable to coordinate them without assistance. I schedule all of his appointments and at the end of the month, email his schedule for the next month to the activities director, rides coordinator, wellness director, and my client. The rides coordinator makes sure all rides are scheduled. The wellness director makes sure the medication list is prepared for the doctor's reference on the day of the appointment. I give notice for any changes to the appointment schedule.

✻ My client has been hospitalized, and before discharge, the facility wellness director visits him to confirm that they will be able to manage his care on his return. Following her assessment, I work with the wellness director and the hospital social worker to make sure that adaptive equipment and home health services are ordered.

✻ A client has accumulated so much stuff that facility housekeeping services are unable to keep the apartment clean and free of trip hazards. My client and I meet with the wellness director who explains the concerns. I assist my client to hire a service to help clear out unneeded possessions and organize what remains. Following, a housekeeping service is hired to supplement the housekeeping services provided by the facility.

Common Problems in Assisted Living and Dementia Care

Food and nutrition

Some days I'm a care manager, and some days I'm a complaint manager. Even the best assisted living and dementia care facilities suffer from staff turnover. While I have sympathy for the often poorly paid and over-stressed staff, my job is to look after the needs of my clients. And even the best facilities can't supply every nutritional need for an aging and often less than healthy clientele.

Many complaints from those in assisted living concern the food. Residents have considerable differences in food preferences as well as in nutritional requirements for healthy aging. So facilities juggle needs, preferences, and variety. Even fine restaurants rarely please every customer, but dissatisfied residents can't take their dining experience elsewhere.

Food problems go beyond the taste buds. Cognitively capable residents can work around a limited menu and make appropriate choices, but those with dementia may make choices that can lead to health problems.

Unlike nursing home personnel, staff in assisted living facilities can't monitor food and fluid intake. A client who makes poor choices that result in weight loss or gain, dehydration, fatigue, or other health problems needs assistance from a combination of doctors, family, and if available, the facility. If I see a problem developing, I request that my client's physician order weekly weight monitoring, a check for vital signs, and sufficient fluids when meds are given.

The resident nurse can direct staff to encourage a resident to choose a balanced meal, but they can't refuse to serve the food clients insist on. Assisted living facilities are required, by law, to support the choices of their residents. Even elders with dementia are responsible for the risk associated with their choices.

As you'll see, below, my success in implementing a change to a client's food habits was mixed. Care facilities have been the arena of my most intransigent challenges.

✻ Bob moved to an assisted living facility after his wife passed away and quickly gained twenty pounds. But after being diagnosed with dementia, his family notices that Bob's food choices narrow, which leads to weight loss.

Every day, Bob orders a bacon, lettuce, and tomato sandwich for lunch, but eats only the bacon. Still hungry, he asks for ice cream. At dinner, after a few bites of his meal, he again has ice cream and takes cookies for a later snack. He eats only toast and coffee for breakfast.

His meal selections leave him with a diet of bacon, toast, ice cream, and cookies. Yum, sure, but not health-sustaining.

The facility nurse modifies Bob's care plan: he will be offered a nutritious alternative to the bacon, lettuce, and tomato sandwich that he takes to mean, *I'll have a BLT, hold the lettuce, hold the tomato, hold the bread.* Unfortunately, unless Bob's friend (and table mate) encourages it, Bob does not go for the offered alternative. At best, when joining him at lunch, Bob's family members choose his meal.

Because of his weight loss, Bob's doctor orders weekly weight and vital signs checks and orders healthy snacks be provided twice a day between meals.

When Bob joins the facility's dementia program, another problem arises. He eats several pastries during the morning program and isn't hungry for lunch. The daily snacks are dropped because Bob won't eat them.

My last suggestion to help Bob is ignored. The dementia program leader serves pastries during his groups. While he moves the pastries from Bob's reach after he has a few, he does not follow my suggestion to replace the pastries with healthy snacks.

✻ Sophie suffers from insulin-dependent diabetes and heart disease. She requires strict adherence to a low-carbohydrate, low-fat, low-salt, no-sugar diet. Although her assisted living facility takes pride in its healthy menu options, for Sophie, the choices are still insufficient. For example, she has to bring her own low-fat and sugar-free salad dressings to meals. Few of the regular menu items meet her requirements, and the facility can't accommodate her while satisfying the majority of the residents. Sophie has to supplement the facility-provided meals with her own condiments and food, which significantly increases her living expenses.

Staff turnover

Moving into a facility is a difficult decision, and your client's ongoing relationships with staff are important. Every facility in which a client of mine has lived has had turnover that's affected their care or well being. To minimize problems that could result from staff turnover, I quickly establish a working relationship with new staff members who will serve my client, and I help my client to do the same.

* I'm hired as care manager for an 82-year-old woman, who, before she hired me, planned a move from one assisted living facility to another. I work with the wellness director of the facility and with my client's attorney-in-fact (AIF) to coordinate the move.

Two weeks after my client moves to the new facility, the wellness director that the AIF and I had been working with resigns his position, and another staff member assumes his responsibilities. Several of the care agreements we made are lost in the transition, which included that my client's personal laundry is to be washed. We don't learn of this oversight until a month has passed, when it's reported that my client has an odor. Although the problem is eventually corrected, in the meantime, my client suffers a reduction in care.

* Before I was hired, a middle-aged client with multiple health issues moved into a retirement/assisted living facility. In the following six years, my role increases from oversight of medical care to coordination of all medical, therapy, and other appointments, and coordination of care provided by the facility. During those six years, my client and I have to deal with five different wellness directors.

Aside from the transition issues—such as consistency of procedures, attention to medication management and care, and involvement in the negotiated care plan review—my client has to adjust to the personalities and styles of the various directors. These directors do more than coordinate care, they also set the tone for staff—how staff performs their duties and how they regard relationships with the residents and their care managers. Given that, with each new director change, I advise my client to inform me of emerging concerns.

With each new director, I have a short conversation and introduce myself as my client's care manager. I make it known I will be monitoring my client's well-being. Unfortunate as it may be, it's human nature to pay extra attention to those who are being especially looked after.

Part VI

Your Career

Chapter 29

How to Have a Career—Private Practice

There's a good chance that none of your previous work or intern experience will prepare you for starting a private practice in care consultation/care management. And you will probably not find solace that you're on similar ground experienced by doctors, lawyers, counselors, physical therapists, and others in the health professions who go into private practice for the first time. Starting a business turns you from an educated trained professional to a novice once again.

I'd like to console you with the choice that you can always join an agency that takes much of the learning to create a practice out of your hands. Lawyers, counselors, physical therapists can, after all, join agencies and focus on just their work. Unfortunately, as a less well-established profession, there aren't many similar opportunities in care consultation/care management, so a career in it might have to be a career in private practice. On the good side, that's also where a good income lies, and there's not nearly as much competition as in other healthcare professions.

I was fortunate to start out in agencies. After several years working with elders in various capacities, I got my first job as a "care manager" in a large agency devoted to serving the elderly and infirm. As I was replacing the retiring Director of Care Management, I believed that the business end of it would be taken care of. I was mistaken. My work for the next five years would combine the disadvantages of being a traditionally low-paid social worker with the novel disadvantage of having to create the equivalent of a private practice within the agency. There was no third-party reimbursement for my services, so I was expected to bring in the income to pay my own salary and then some. For five years, I had to counter the agency's tradition of providing free service (reimbursed by third parties), by building a private-pay practice within.[1]

The situation at the agency was not without advantages. We landed a crisis clinic contract where I would be paid for ten hours per referral to work with the family care givers of elders and the disabled. As my paid time with these clients was restricted, and most often moderate to low-income clients made use of the service, my work with them would be limited—that is, I would not become their care manager. My task was to arrange services for these clients they could afford in the long term. It was in this situation that I began to learn much of what would become useful as a care consultant. I learned to work efficiently, with the dual goals of alleviating problems with elders, while doing so as frugally for them as possible.

My work with the crisis clinic might be the best training I had for private practice. Many agencies and practitioners of a service believe that the best way to earn a living is to maximize the financial gain from each opportunity. In contrast, I believe much of my success comes from giving clients the best value—that my work may not just contribute to their health and well being, but also ultimately to their bank account. For example, my services complement that of a lawyer when I'm both

[1]Anyone trained in social work will have to overcome the *volunteer* orientation that translates to *service should be free*—commonplace for agency social work.

cheaper and more suitable for those situations. I get many referrals from lawyers for that reason. I know the appropriate services, and I know the providers of those services that have proved to be competent and trustworthy.

Networking

One of my early mistakes in private practice was that I believed I would get most of my referrals from other care managers and those who focus on problems of the elderly. My mantra at networking meetings was that there are an abundance of clients, and we'd refer to each other along the lines of our special expertise.

It's an understatement that I was being näive, or a social worker—same thing. It's not easy to earn a living in social services; most of us aren't driving a Mercedes. The inclination is to not share, but to hold on to a client or potential client like it's the last Cheeto at a Super Bowl party.

Once again, a successful practice comes from solving the problems of others, but not just from solving the problems of clients and their families. By being the best care manager to whom they can refer, a successful practice also comes from solving the problems of other professionals. When a lawyer, doctor, accountant, crisis clinic, elder service, and others can't serve the care needs of an elder, I can provide a service to those professionals as well as to the elders and their families.

The approximate order of my referral sources have been lawyers, the listings in professional organizations to which I belong, doctors, previous clients and their families, random agencies, and on rare occasions, other care managers.

I have no secret to networking. Sending out brochures to local lawyers has yielded somewhere between zero and no referrals. Mixing at conferences hasn't done much for my practice: no one there cares about my payment for the Toyota Corolla on the 5th of the month; they're thinking about their own monthly overhead. As with most successful networking, word-of-mouth and doing great work is the gold standard.[2] Build your reputation by being good at taking problems off the hands of both other professionals and your clients' families.

Referrals

Damn it! Jim! I'm a doctor not a . . .
—Bones McCoy (a character from the original Star Trek)

I get annoyed by inappropriate referrals because these referrals (by nature of them being inappropriate) are time-consuming but do nothing for my practice. Typically, they require a referral to a mental health, social service, or other agency, many of which I have little knowledge. Just as any other non-expert must do, I search the Web.

My annoyance stems from knowing that the referrers are being lazy, just finding someone to pass the inquiring customer to without attempting to really help. No one appreciates being passed around, so regardless that it takes attention from my own practice, I make an effort to find the right match.

Unless I'm having a very bad no good day, it takes but a moment to recognize that my annoyance is stupid and inappropriate. The cost of getting appropriate referrals is getting inappropriate ones. You want referring parties to think of you as often as possible. If my name pops into their heads any time they think elder problem, I'm going to get appropriate referrals more often than not. Get over it, I remind myself, a few minutes of pro bono work is not a hardship.

[2] I'm speaking in metaphors; there's no gold in care consultation, just an interesting career while earning a living.

Ideally, all referrals would be a perfect match for your services.[3] That would mean that you're doing an excellent job of educating lawyers, doctors, eldercare agencies, and other referral sources to understand exactly what you do. Bonus points if you've demonstrated that you do it better than others.

Good referrals

Early in my career, I worked in a crisis clinic that operated out of the psychiatric ward. On occasion, I'd be called to interview someone who arrived in the emergency room of the hospital, across the street. On one of my visits, an emergency room doctor told me that he could never do what I did. And I replied that I could never do what he did. Excellent. We both have careers because we take on the other's burden. When you've given referral sources enough to understand your work, either through information or—much better—through experience with you, you're in a position to take a burden off their hands. We all have things we're not good at or just dislike. Good referrals—and by that I mean, they actually need *your* services, and they actually contact you for a consultation—usually happen when you're taking on someone else's burden.[4]

Not-so-good referrals

Stop me if you've heard this one. A telemarketer calls with bad news: your services are in demand, but clients can't find you because you're not listed with their (expensive) listing service. The burden you're being asked to take off their hands is different from the one I described above. These marketers want you to take on the burden of their insufficient income.

[3] Ideally, all your referrals to other services would be a perfect match.

[4] By "burden," I mean the responsibility to find the best resource for someone in need.

A rule of thumb is that if you get a referral from advertising, you're going to get lesser quality referrals—window-shoppers, people seeking free advice (if they expect several lengthy phone calls to explain their issues, before they hire you, they probably won't), and those who don't have the authority to hire you on someone else's behalf. Occasionally, you'll get a sincere client from an ad, but don't make that the cornerstone of your marketing.

In a nutshell, here's how to have a career: be just the right service to help a client, and do all that you can to educate potential referral sources what it is you do—especially, what you do better than their other sources. Help the referring person feel good that they know the perfect choice and help them make that choice you.

Your Tools—Phone, Computer, and Office

There are things I absolutely don't believe, anymore. I no longer believe in Santa Claus. I no longer believe in the tooth fairy. I no longer believe in the sanity of political campaigns.

And there are things that I still barely believe. I barely believe that I used to drive 40 minutes to an office merely to use a desk phone. I barely believe that I used to drive 40 minutes to an office to use a desk computer. I barely believe that I used to stop at various public phone booths to make appointments and other business calls on-the-go. Sheesh.

I'm one of those people who lament the ubiquity of high tech in our lives. While my husband and adult children attend steadily to their smart phones, as if concerned, any moment, their iPhones will disappear in The Rapture for Apple Devices, I'm applying similar devotion to the vegetation, soil, and feathered visitors in my garden. But boy is my life better for high tech.

My firstborn cell phone weighed nearly as much as my firstborn child, but it was the beginning of my vocational liberation. Still working for an agency, I persuaded my boss to have a virtual private network (no, I don't know what that means, but the description is encouraging) installed in my home office. As I was able to be far more efficient, my life got a lot better, and my employer got more for their money. Currently, seventy percent of my consultation and management is done by phone, and (as the joke goes) the other seventy percent is done on my iPad. I'm someone who always prefers face-to-face communication, but since much of my work is acting as a liaison among healthcare professionals, facilities, family members, and otherwise involved, I'm usually making and fielding calls, or exchanging email.

I choose my tools (to be fair, I make my business partner, who happens to be my husband, choose my tools, while I'm busy in the garden) to be light, reliable, and to be as easy to use as possible. My car, phone, and computer are all IRS-recognized business expenses and are cheap compared to the tools needed in most other businesses.

Most of my work is done either in my home office or on-the-go in clients' homes, assisted living facilities, hospitals, and doctors' and dentists' offices. But I still have a business office where I meet new clients and involved family members for consultation sessions. I probably average less than ten hours a month in this office, but I still find it necessary. Meeting in a public space results in privacy issues and distractions. Where office space is expensive, I know practitioners who rent part-time space on designated days of the week. A small conference room, as long as it's completely private, can work.

If you feel you're fighting the very tools that you've chosen to make your work life easier, don't blame yourself, blame the tools. If they're not working for you, there are other solutions.

Chapter 30

How to Have a Career—Money, Theirs

Care management is not, currently, recognized as a healthcare service, so my work is not covered by Medicare or other health insurance.[1] As when hiring lawyers, accountants, and palm readers, my services must be paid for by the client. As we know, those without means can't afford lawyers, accountants, and often, palm readers. And while many can't afford care manager services, one of the advantages of hiring a care manager is that they can save clients money.

Ethics

One of the practices a professional can do is to refer to a lower-cost provider. For example, physicians can refer to physical therapists, psychologists, or masters-level clinicians; accountants can refer to bookkeepers or an online service; and lawyers can refer to paralegals and care managers.

[1] I will be surprised if care management is ever covered by health insurance.

I have established a relationship with a number of lawyers. We don't compete in the services space, we complement the other's work. Clients save money when their lawyers decide that my services are appropriate. In turn, clients save money when I decide that, for example, a care provider, placement specialist, or counselor can provide a less expensive service than I can.

Ethical dilemmas that aren't

Another consideration for a care manager is their clients' assets versus their quality of life. Clients with the means can have their lives enhanced in a variety of ways. Some of my clients have had more money than they could ever spend, but my unnecessary concerns for their finances kept me from recommending additional life-enhancing services. This is another example of making it clear in your mind whether decisions are for your needs or for that of the client. Just because I'm frugal doesn't mean I should be frugal for my clients when it's unwarranted.

The elephant in the assisted living facility

Nearly all the relatives who stood to inherit money from my clients have acted with love and caring rather than greed. Nearly. The concerns of loved ones responsible for making financial decisions on my clients' behalf have usually been about making the money last as long as necessary. But (as I've stated more than once), on occasion, the concern has been about hoarding unspent money the relatives would inherit. That's one of the toughest issues a care manager will deal with because it will always be left unsaid. Who's going to say aloud, "We don't want that for her because we want the money after she dies"?

While I'm a relentless advocate of my client, I'm not anyone's family therapist, so I see no advantage in challenging anyone's motives for their financial decisions. I work around things left unsaid as best I can, primarily, by emphasizing cost-saving approaches to getting my client appropriate services.

As I've said, I believe that I provide value, and often, money-saving expertise. And I try to make my services as cost-effective as possible, for example, by combining client visits in a way that minimizes travel-time billing. However, if you don't value what you offer, then don't expect anyone else to. I'm fair, I'm efficient, and I charge for my services.

Chapter 31

How to Have a Career—Money, Yours

When I was thirteen, for some unfathomable reason, I decided to become a social worker. That budding adolescent stage was the only time I ever planned my career. I certainly hadn't intended to work with elders. The years that followed earning my MSW, I worked in mental health. My move to working with elders was by chance. I moved to a small town, where the only opening for a social worker in the local counseling agency was as Geriatric Program Coordinator. The work with elders fit me, and I went on to hold similar positions in other agencies.

At the time, unlike clinical social work, care management was not widely recognized as a distinct service. The responsibility of care management was spread around to an agency social worker, medical staff, and family members. The problem and failure of that approach is that the heart of care management is coordinating care, and multiple managers equals no managers. In a position that was regarded much like an unidentified flying object, I had to make myself and services known to referral sources, clients, and too often, coworkers.

As I stated previously, in my agency positions, I was in circumstances that many would view as the worst of both worlds. Within an agency that charged health insurance for their other services, I had to create a private-pay business. I took on an entrepreneurial challenge with a cog-in-a-machine salary. It was like going into private practice without the financial upside. After some years of nagging from my husband (Did I say nagging? I meant gentle encouragement), I went into private practice.

While I sometimes resented my worst-of-both-worlds situation at the agency, I benefited through the experience in creating a practice. Still, now completely on my own, I had to learn to run an office, bill clients, manage accounting records, keep client records secure, and maintain office insurance and professional insurance.

Our Business Solutions—Your Solutions May Vary

Lawyers and accountants are trained and qualified to give, respectively, legal and accounting counsel. We are not. The following describes solutions that work for us. We have no idea whether our solutions will work for you. *We provide an example, not advice.*

Also, federal and state regulations change, so anything that follows can be stale by the time you read it.

Records and billing

I've found no convenient packaged solutions for professionals who handle healthcare records but do not bill third parties. Online billing services that deal with health care are designed to facilitate medical insurance billing—specifically, to make diagnoses and reimbursement submissions relatively easy, and to make the handling of healthcare related data ("protected health information") HIPAA compliant. As my business takes only private pay, I find online billing services that deal with health care to be cluttered with services I don't use. Nevertheless, if I were starting now in private practice, regardless of the overkill and expense of online medical billing services, I would consider one. These services not only provide billing, but if you're willing to type all your notes online, they also provide records security and (often) secure email. I find private practice demanding enough without dealing with security and privacy issues.

I've rolled my own solutions through desktop billing software, encrypted local storage, encrypted local backup, and handwritten notes that I keep in a locked file cabinet in a locked room—in other words, the old-fashioned way. I also back up my records digitally; I scan them on a lightning-fast Fuji SnapScan and upload them to a HIPAA compliant cloud service.[1] That way, I'm covered if I have a fire or unfriendly visit from Godzilla.

Nuts and Bolts

Business entities and taxes

Because we (the business is owned by Gary and me) once dabbled in Web services, and wanted some liability shielding for our *non-professional* services, we formed a Limited Liability Company (LLC), rather than a sole proprietorship. For just the care consultation services, because an LLC does not shield us from liability for our healthcare-related professional services, we'd have gone with a sole proprietorship. We get our professional liability insurance through our professional organizations. We would not practice without it.

In my state (maybe all, dunno), any business entity can apply for an assumed name. Because I don't want checks written to my business to be refused for deposit, I accept checks under my business name, Aging Well LLC, and several assumed names,[2] which I obtained for a small fee

[1]Whether you need a HIPAA compliant service is up to you and your lawyer.
[2]Assumed names are also often called *doing business as*, or DBAs for short.

through my state government. For example, I can deposit checks written to Aging Well LLC, Aging Well, Joan McGinnis MSW, and Joan McGinnis.

Banking

When I applied for a business bank account in the name of Aging Well LLC, the bank required proof of my business name and the Employee Identification Number (EIN) that was issued to me by the U.S. Treasury (IRS).[3]

I considered getting a business credit card from our bank until I learned that, if I apply for a business credit card, I'm really applying for a business loan. Apparently, I should have kept better records of my childhood lemonade stand. Instead, to keep track of business expenses, I just use a separate credit card.[4]

[3]https://www.irs.gov/businesses/small-businesses-self-employed/employer-id-numbers

[4]I could use a business debit card, but I was spooked when I learned that consumer protection laws don't apply to business accounts.

Chapter 32

Conclusion

If you've read this far, you've probably developed an idea of whether a career in this field is right for you. Do you have and relish the traits essential for this work? Do you have compassion for the frail and elderly; deep respect for their life experiences; emotional toughness to advocate for your clients nonstop and deal with the death of many of them; fortitude to face the complexity in healthcare systems, legal systems, family systems, care agency and residential systems; and finally, in addition to your primary work with elders and their families, the self-reliance to run a business in all that entails—as a marketer, bookkeeper, and office manager?

If you're old enough to consider becoming a care consultant, you've already encountered many learning challenges: You've learned to negotiate your familial and social worlds through the many stages of growing up. You've learned to drive a car—a complex physical and mental skill you now employ by second nature. Most of you have learned to negotiate (for sure, with varying success) intimate relationships, and some of you have raised or are raising children. You also likely have learned a complex hobby, musical instrument, and/or a vocation.

Even with those prior successes, it's difficult to learn something new that has lots of parts, lots of systems. We learn complex pursuits from the inside out, one experience at a time. We integrate these experiences to face the next professional challenge with improved confidence. That's as good as it gets.

We've given aspiring care consultants a head start by describing my professional experience. We've passed along a mix of knowledge and conveyed an attitude, an attitude of compassion and respect towards your future clientele, but one that allows each care consultant to construct his or her own practice.

We welcome thoughtful praise and criticism (though we prefer praise) on Amazon and other book review sites.

Write us at
Joan@JoanMcGinnisMSW.com
GeBloom@iCloud.com

Subscribe to online updates to the book and be notified of future products from Aging Well Press: AgingWell.us/AgingWellPress

Acknowledgements

The authors thank our friend and colleague, Brad Lancaster, for his significant contributions to our book, some with his name on it, some disguised with fake mustache and glasses. We also thank our friend and colleague, Denise Hie, who spotted typos and poorly formed sentences. We forgive both of them for ruining our illusion of perfection.

Joan also thanks Cecilia London and Nora Gibson, who helped Joan get started on her career in care consultation and care management.

While we acknowledge the assistance, Joan and Gary made final decisions on all content, grammar, spelling, formatting, cover design, typefaces, and everything else but the chemical and engineering process that created the object we call a book. In short, the responsibility for this work lies entirely with the authors.

Index